Praise for *The Whole Heart Solution* and Joel K. Kahn, MD

"If you want to raise your heart energy, keep your heart arteries clean, and identify the root causes of heart disease to avoid stents and bypass surgery, Dr. Kahn has your prescriptions ready to use. This is a unique manual of caring for your heart by taking out the bad stuff and putting in the good stuff. A must-read."

—Mark Hyman, MD, *New York Times* bestselling author of *UltraMetabolism, Blood Sugar Solution,* and others

"Our medical care system is broken and the only way to fix it is by teaching Americans how to protect themselves against disease to avoid medical care. Invasive cardiology is a billion dollar industry based on disproven science. Coronary artery disease and heart attacks are avoidable through superior nutrition. Dr. Kahn can lead the way to change the face of cardiology in America."

—Joel Fuhrman, MD, *New York Times* bestselling author of *Eat to Live, The End of Diabetes* and others

"Coronary artery disease is not a 'disease,' but a survival mechanism. Basically, our body is trying to survive our lifestyle. It is about time that a cardiologist of the caliber of Dr. Kahn writes a book to educate both patients and doctors how to avoid stenting blocked arteries."

—Alejandro Junger, MD, *New York Times* bestselling author of *Clean*

"Dr. Joel Kahn is a functional medicine rock star! His book provides a critical guide for every patient with heart disease and those who want to avoid it. Dr. Kahn brilliantly uncovers the true root causes and treatments of cardiovascular disease, making the complex simple to understand and even easier to apply. I know Dr. Kahn well, and his life, passion and medical work will ensure that this book will be widely read and change lives everywhere."

—Tana Amen, BSN, RN, author of the *Brain Doctor's Wife* series and *OmniDiet*

"This is an important book that everyone needs to read. Heart disease and brain disease are intimately connected. Your brain uses 20 percent of the blood flow in your brain. If your heart is troubled it increases your risk of depression and dementia. Dr. Kahn is an expert at translating complex information into easy to understand, usable techniques to have a better heart and brain."

—Daniel G. Amen, MD, *New York Times* bestselling author of *Change Your Brain, Change Your Life* and others

"Lifestyle changes can effectively cure the #1 killer in the industrialized world. That's why a book like this is so critical. Hundreds of thousands of lives hang in the balance."

—Michael Greger, MD, bestselling author of *Carbophobia*

"Dr. Joel Kahn's book will give you the reasons 'why' all our hearts are in danger and necessary 'how' for self transformation. As a passionate leader of health and wellness Dr. Kahn demonstrates how heart disease cannot be compartmentalized and is related to the whole person. Like the man himself, this is a book that will first open your heart and then heal it."

—Jonny Kest, founder of Center for Yoga and national director of yoga, Lifetime Fitness Corporation

"Dr. Joel Kahn is a leader in the cardiology world in recognizing the importance of food and lifestyle for heart conditions. Credible doctors like Dr. Kahn, who are not only expert in high-tech medicine but also have an interest and knowledge in holistic approaches, are rare. His book will be a winner for all involved."

> —Neal D. Barnard, MD, bestselling author of *Dr. Neal Barnard's Program for Reversing Diabetes*

"Dr. Joel Kahn, a leader in preventive cardiology, [offers] provocative insights, a deep well of knowledge, and a clear view of the big picture. When someone trained to put stents into occluded coronary arteries is prepared to tell us how to avoid that fate, we should all pay close attention! I will certainly be sharing this book with all of my patients."

> —David Katz, MD, Director, Preventive Medicine at Yale University and author of *Disease Proof*

"Dr. Joel Kahn has a national reputation as one of the top cardiologists in the U.S. [His book] will be a tremendous asset to patients, their families and physicians."

> —Mark Houston, MD, MS, Director, Hypertension Institute and Vascular Biology of Nashville, TN, and author of *What Your Doctor May Not Tell You about Heart Disease*

"*The Whole Heart Solution* by Dr. Joel Kahn is an enlightened and comprehensive examination by a dedicated physician, as well as a treasure chest of opportunities to enhance a full and healthy life."

> —Caldwell B. Esselstyn, Jr., MD, author of *Prevent and Reverse Heart Disease*

"Dr. Kahn is the rare breed that has both traditional medical training of the highest quality and a keen interest and expertise in food as medicine, stress management, and nutrition and supplements. In my work as a healing chef, I know that much progress needs to be made in preventing heart disease. I know that my friend Dr. Joel Kahn will achieve that in this book."

> —Tal Ronnen, author of *The Conscious Cook* and Executive Chef, Wynn Hotels, Las Vegas

"The heart can be strengthened in so many ways without sugery. Doctors need to be champions of real health, food-based health, fitness-based health. I know champions, and Dr. Kahn is a champion."

> —John Salley, four-time NBA champ

"Dr. Joel Kahn is one of the foremost cardiologists in America today. His natural approach to preventing and/or curing heart disease [presented in] this book is a powerful and practical tool for bestowing vitality and longevity."

> —James O'Keefe, MD, Director of Preventive Cardiology at Mid America Heart Institute and bestselling author of *The Forever Young Diet and Lifestyle*

"Dr. Kahn is a champion of health and a persuasive catalyst for lifestyle transformation. His book will inspire and equip many to lead a more healthy life."

> —Dee Eastman, Director of *The Daniel Plan* at Saddleback Church

"As a vegan chef, I appreciate Dr. Kahn's well-researched efforts to encourage a plant based diet to reduce heart disease and diabetes. Few doctors have the courage to direct their patients down this path."

> —George Vutetakis, author of *Vegetarian Traditions*

THE Whole Heart SOLUTION

HALT HEART DISEASE NOW WITH THE BEST ALTERNATIVE AND TRADITIONAL MEDICINE

JOEL K. KAHN, MD

Preventive Cardiologist and Clinical Professor of Medicine
at Wayne State University School of Medicine

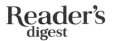

The Reader's Digest Association, Inc.
New York, NY/Montreal

A READER'S DIGEST BOOK

Copyright © 2013 Joel K. Kahn, MD

All rights reserved. Unauthorized reproduction, in any manner, is prohibited.

Reader's Digest is a registered trademark of The Reader's Digest Association, Inc.

The Library of Congress has catalogued the original edition of this book as follows:

Kahn, Joel K.
  Holistic heart book: a preventive cardiologist's guide to halt heart disease now / Joel K. Kahn, MD.
     pages cm
  Includes bibliographical references and index.
  ISBN 978-1-62145-143-3 (alk. paper) -- ISBN 978-1-62145-151-8 (epub)
  1. Heart--Diseases--Alternative treatment. 2. Holistic medicine. I. Title.
  RC684.A48H65 2013
  616.1'205--dc23

                     2013040399

We are committed to both the quality of our products and the service we provide to our customers. We value your comments, so please feel free to contact us.

The Reader's Digest Association, Inc.

Adult Trade Publishing

44 South Broadway

White Plains, NY 10601

For more Reader's Digest products and information, visit our website:

www.rd.com (in the United States)

www.readersdigest.ca (in Canada)

Printed in the United States of America

3 5 7 9 10 8 6 4 2

NOTE TO OUR READERS

Dedication

I dedicate this book to my father, Irwin L. Kahn, and my father-in-law, Arthur J. Fischer, MD, both of blessed memory. My father's strong and creative personality formed many of my views and opinions. During his 25 years as a heart patient, he was an early follower of the Pritikin Longevity Center's program. My father-in-law took me on hospital rounds when I was in high school and helped me fall in love with caring for patients as if they were my best friends.

Contents

Acknowledgments

For several decades, my wife, Karen, has been urging me to write a book. When I finally decided to follow her suggestion, I assumed the process would be easy. And it was, or so I thought. I sat down and wrote a book in just a few weeks. Little did I know that my initial rough draft was only the first step in a very long, multistep process.

I've been fortunate. An incredible team of talented people has supported me and helped me to improve on my initial effort. I am eternally grateful.

Thanks to my friends Daniel Amen, MD, and Tana Amen, RN, BSN. During lunch at a medical meeting during the fall of 2012, Dr. Amen gladly shared his many insights into the publishing process. His advice proved to be sage. Tana has been a supporter and colleague since the day I met her at a medical meeting in the winter of 2011. To this day I feel lucky to call her a dear friend.

Thanks to all of my teachers, including William O'Neill, James Willerson, David Hillis, Geoffrey Hartzler, and Barry Rutherford. When I went back to university in 2011 to study metabolic cardiology, I was grateful for the guidance of Drs. Howard Wright, Pamela Smith, Mark Houston, Mimi Guarneri, James Roberts, Joe Lamb, Deanna Minich, and Jeffrey Bland.

A special thanks goes to Lisa Hagan, my amazing literary agent and my most vocal supporter. You have been so incredible at helping me move from concept to completion.

A big thanks also goes to Jason Wochub and Kerry Shaw of MindBodyGreen.com for giving me the opportunity to write on health matters weekly and form my message to the public.

The team at *Reader's Digest*, headed by senior editor Andrea

Au Levitt in the book publishing group and senior editor Lauren Gelman at the magazine, has made this project so easy. I was steered to them for a reason, and it has been a pleasure to work with them from day one. Alisa Bowman, who has come to share my passion for health and prevention, has polished a rough stone to make it what I hope you feel is now a sparkling jewel.

My mother, Ruth Kahn, has been an advocate of healthy living for decades. Her transition from Hungarian goulash to quinoa and lentil dinners, her commitment to self-education, and her amazing focus on exercise including Zumba classes even now into her early 80s has helped shape and support me. I love you.

To my children, Daniel, Jacob, and Jessica, and Daniel's wife Yany, who have provided love and support and who have willingly tried strange healthy food in our travels all over the world.

Finally, to my wife, Karen. In our marriage of over 30 years, if I took a step toward something new, she stepped right along with me and often took the lead. With her nursing education and her recent completion of training as a health and nutrition educator, she has always been my biggest supporter, resource, and lifemate. I love you.

Part One

Whole Heart Facts

We can't see our hearts, but we can feel them beating. Perhaps you can feel your own heart lightly thumping away in your chest right now. How long this fist-sized muscle will continue to send blood and nutrients to all of the parts of your body depends on the fuel you feed it, as well as how well you care for all of your cells, tissues, and organs. Yes, it takes an entire body to keep a heart beating, and that's why the prescriptions in *The Whole Heart Solution* will help you maintain total body health, not just the health of your heart.

In this section, you'll come to understand why holistic heart health is so important, discover important tools and tests to assess your complete heart health status, and learn why natural remedies such as diet, fitness, and stress relief are often just as effective (and in some cases more so) than many state-of-the-art medications and invasive procedures.

It's my hope that this knowledge will motivate you to incorporate the dozens of whole heart prescriptions you will find in Part Two of this book.

Chapter 1

My Prescription for a Lasting Heart

As I stood at the front of a giant circular auditorium in the basement of the medical school, I stared for a moment at 250 young faces. These future physicians sat with open laptops, waiting for me to say my first word.

"I can't believe what I'm *not* going to tell them," I thought.

I was about to deliver a lecture on *preventive* cardiology to the second-year students at Wayne State University School of Medicine, the largest medical school in America. These medical students had been taught what to do after heart disease had already set in. They were well educated in techniques such as determining cholesterol-lowering medications, stenting, and even bypass surgery. They knew how to take an electrocardiogram, as well as how to interpret the results.

But how to ensure a patient never ends up in a cardiologist's office in the first place? This had never been taught.

It was an important moment, and I was thrilled that the medical school had made such a historic change in curriculum and had tapped me, a clinical professor of medicine at the school, to help put that change into effect. Still, in the weeks leading up to the big day, I'd fretted. How would I ever find a way to condense everything I knew about preventing heart disease into a lecture that lasted not even one hour?

For these students to pass their examinations and boards, they needed to know how risk factors like diabetes, high blood pressure, and high blood cholesterol cause arteries to harden, clog, and narrow. That alone would take up the entire time I'd been allotted, and yet, what about the causes behind the causes? What about food toxins that irritate the linings of the arteries, causing them to harden and set the stage for high blood pressure? How would I ever express how the health of every part of the body—including the lungs, the gums, the digestive tract, and even the sex organs—affects heart health? What about how everything from air pollution to poor sleep to plastic bottles to stress affects our cells and, by proxy, our hearts, too?

"Fifty minutes is a good start, but it's not nearly enough time," I thought, and then I began talking.

The Whole Heart Solution covers what I would have taught those medical students if I'd had free rein—four or five hours of lecture time—and faculty support to rewrite medical textbooks. It includes dozens of prescriptions that will help you make sure your heart lasts a very long time. These prescriptions are probably not at all like the kinds you've previously received from your health care provider. None require a trip to a drugstore, and you might find many of them quite surprising. For instance, one of my prescriptions recommends you read the ingredients label on your toothpaste. Another will have you counting your blessings. Still another suggests you try walking barefoot. You might wonder: What do such practices have to do with preventing heart disease? The answer is, everything.

Still, despite hundreds of medical research studies and anecdotal support for the importance and effectiveness of every single one of the prescriptions in this book, this information is not covered in medical school or recommended by health care professionals, and much of it has slipped past the notice of the media, too.

With this book, it's my hope that these important prescriptions don't escape your notice as well.

No matter your current state of health, the recommendations you'll find within the pages of this book can help make sure your heart keeps beating long into your old age. If you are still healthy and reading this book in hopes of escaping a family history of the world's number one killer, you'll find what you need to know to do just that. If you've already been diagnosed with high cholesterol, high blood sugar, or high blood pressure, there's still time to put these suggestions to work.

If you suffer from angina (chest pain) or have undergone stenting or bypass surgery, incorporating these recommendations can halt the progression of your heart disease and possibly even reverse it.

No matter where you are on the heart disease continuum, it's not too early and it's not too late.

THE KILLER YOU DON'T WANT TO MEET

That day, when I stood in front of those medical students, I said what I will now tell you: It's more important for you to prevent and treat heart and blood vessel diseases such as stroke than any other illnesses.

Heart disease kills many more people than Alzheimer's disease.

It brings an untimely end to more lives than airline crashes and car accidents.

It's the same even with terrorism and violent crime.

Do you find this surprising? Do you think about heart disease whenever you take a bite of food in the same way, for instance, you might think about life and death whenever a plane lifts off the runway?

If you are like most people, the answer is probably no. Indeed, if you haven't been diagnosed with a heart condition, and, if you are like the vast majority of people I know, you probably don't think about heart disease much at all until the tragedy strikes. Rather, the disease that plagues your thoughts is one that is less likely to end your life: cancer.

According to the World Health Organization, heart disease kills more people in high-income countries than any cancer multiplied by three. That's right: One-third of all deaths around the world stem from heart disease, and only 12 percent from cancer.[1]

These are mothers and fathers, brothers and sisters, spouses and children, friends and coworkers, clergy and health care workers who suffer heart attacks, strokes, and blood vessel diseases at an alarming frequency. That's a lot of lives cut much too short, and, sadly, three-quarters of those deaths could have been prevented, but not in the ways you might suspect such as bypass surgery.

In the past few decades, we've experienced dramatic improvements in medical care. The pharmaceutical industry has brought us miracle medicines capable of halving the amount of blood cholesterol floating around in our arteries. Along with my colleagues, I have perfected ways to thread the tiniest of catheters into a coronary artery and insert medicine-coated stents to hold it open and allow blood to flow. Robots have even been invented to help with the trickiest aspects of open-heart surgery.

But despite these advances in medical care, far too many people are dying years or decades before their time. More than one million coronary bypass and angioplasty surgeries are done every single year in the United States and Canada, making these procedures among the most expensive and most common medical procedures offered in North America.[2] Still, no other cause of death has even come close to ousting heart disease from its number one spot on the list of the top 10 killers of men and women worldwide.

I tell you none of this to scare you. Rather, as a compassionate cardiologist, I wrote this book because I want you to know something both important and liberating. You do not need to get sick. You also don't need to have your chest cracked open so a surgeon can sew veins onto your diseased coronary arteries. You don't need to suffer from side effects of your medications, and you definitely don't need to be disabled or die from heart disease decades before your time.

You have so much more control over this killer than you think—almost total control, in fact.

But your first step lies in taking this killer seriously. Most people don't. They instead focus on the wrong health priorities. They say a prayer as a plane lifts off a runway, but they never think twice about the possible health ramifications of sitting still during that multihour flight while they consume highly processed snack foods. They've undergone so many mammograms, colon checks, and prostate exams that they've lost count. Yet not only have they never undergone heart CT calcium scoring or advanced cholesterol testing, had the medial thickness of their carotid arteries measured by ultrasound, or had an EndoPAT, they've never even heard of such tests, and that's because their health care providers haven't mentioned them.

Sadly, early detection and prevention of heart disease is not typically taught to medical students, it's often not paid for by insurers, and is usually not practiced by medical doctors, either.

Tell me if this makes sense to you: You go to your medical doctor for a checkup at age 50. You get a recommendation to be screened for colon cancer and you have a colonoscopy that may result in a bill for thousands of dollars. If you are a woman, your health care provider discusses your risk of breast cancer with you, does an exam, and sends you for a mammogram, digital thermography, an ultrasound, or even an MRI. This also costs hundreds and even thousands of dollars.

But colon and breast cancer combined kill far fewer people than heart disease. In comparison, three of the most important screening tools for heart disease (the calcium scoring, EndoPAT, and measurement of carotid artery thickness that I mentioned earlier) are almost never offered, and insurers often won't cover them anyway in most states. Cheaper tests—such as routine blood work and electrocardiograms (ECGs)—are being offered instead. Well, you get what you pay for. These tests often do little to uncover hidden heart disease. Instead they give you and your health care provider a very misleading picture of the state of your arteries. As a result, people with heart disease often end up being told that they have a clean bill of health. They then put most thoughts about heart disease prevention away. They feel little to no motivation to change their lifestyle until their heart disease has progressed far beyond the silent stage.

And then once the heart disease is so rampant that they feel chest pain or shortness of breath, they wonder, "Why didn't anyone catch this sooner?"

That's a shame, and it doesn't have to be this way.

WHAT BREAKS OUR HEARTS

During my short presentation that day at Wayne State University School of Medicine, I mentioned many of the statistics I just shared. I also told those students about the well-known causes of heart disease.

I told those students that I graduated from medical school 30 years ago, and, back then, I was taught that the causes of heart disease had been identified in a famous study about a town in Massachusetts. The Framingham Study began in 1948 and examined all members of this city west of Boston. The findings were profound: High blood pressure, smoking, high cholesterol, age, diabetes mellitus, and a family history of premature heart disease predicted heart disease. Now, three decades later, the same data and approach are still being taught, but we are no closer to saving lives. If anything, we're further away than ever from helping people.

Each year the American Heart Association, the Centers for Disease Control and Prevention, and the National Institutes of Health compile an extensive report that includes the latest heart disease statistics. A quick look at the 2013 report on adults in the United States is enough to make anyone's heart ache:[3]

* 34 percent are obese.

* 13 percent have blood cholesterol levels above 240 milligrams per deciliter (mg/dl).

* 33 percent have high blood pressure.

* 8 percent have diabetes, a condition that doubles their chances of eventually developing heart disease.

* 38 percent have prediabetes and 34 percent have metabolic syndrome (a cluster of health problems that includes obesity and insulin resistance).

The statistics for Canada and many other countries are only slightly better. These diseases all raise your risk for heart disease, and they are *all* preventable.

We know, for instance, some of the causes of obesity: too much sitting coupled with too much eating, particularly of nutrient-poor processed junk foods and drinks. We've known this for many years and yet in developed countries, we're moving in the wrong direction. Among U.S. children aged 18 and younger, 17 percent of girls and 10 percent of boys engage in no physical activity at all, and 32 percent of adults admit that they do not exercise either. In Canada, researchers recently found that the majority of adults spend 68 percent of their waking hours sitting or lying down. That's nearly 10 hours of sitting time a day, and it doesn't include the seven or eight hours they are asleep at night.[4]

And not only are we sitting more, we're eating more. Between 1971 and 2004 (the most current statistics available), U.S. women began consuming, on average, 22 percent more calories (going from 1,500 to 1,800) and men 10 percent more (from 2,400 to 2,600). A recent report also found that Canadians consume about 20 percent of their total calories—one-fifth of all the food they consume—in the form of one food: sugar.[5]

This trend is echoed worldwide. According to the World Health Organization, in the 1960s, the average person consumed 2,300 calories a day. Now, five decades later, the average person in the average developed country consumes 600 more calories than that every single day.[6]

We're eating too much, and we're moving too little. No wonder so many of us are gaining weight. But that's obvious, and, I'm guessing, it's something you already knew.

Here's what's not so obvious. Did you know that common everyday products—such as the moisturizer you use on your skin—might, in part, be behind this surge of obesity, as well as heart disease? Or that some of the foods you might be eating every day—foods you might consider "heart healthy"—contain toxins that erode the lining of your arteries? And here's another one that not many people know: There's a sweet spot when it comes to exercise. Too little may damage your heart, but so may too much.

Those are just three of scores of surprises you'll find within the pages of this book. There are many more ways to prevent heart disease than those identified by the pioneering Framingham researchers. Dozens of ways, in fact. More exciting: Most of these causes are as easy to overcome as changing your breathing pattern, walking a little faster, and making the most of the commercial breaks that play on your TV.

The vast majority of people who suffer from heart attacks, strokes, and other heart-related deaths don't need to suffer at all. *More than 75 percent of heart disease diagnoses could have been prevented.*[7] If they'd only known these prescriptions earlier, these patients wouldn't have needed their stents. They could have gone without their bypass surgeries, too. Many of them probably wouldn't have needed their medications, either, and they definitely didn't need to suffer heart attacks or strokes.

Many of them could still be alive.

It might be too late for them, but it's not too late for you.

In the pages of this book, you'll find a few prescriptions that you can use right away—in the next few minutes—to bring health and vitality to your heart. If you incorporate others, you'll be well on your way to living a heart-healthy lifestyle in as little as a week. If you are diligent about them, you can use my suggestions for more than just preventing heart disease; if you've already experienced any type of a heart-related problem, these suggestions can usually halt any progression. And, if you adopt enough of them, you can even use them to reverse heart disease and grow younger.

The secret to preventing and reversing everyone's number one killer lies in the smallest of decisions you make from the moment you wake until the moment you call it quits for the day. The decisions you make with your fork, your grocery list, your feet, your alarm clock, your social calendar, your personal habits, and much more can all affect your risk of developing or reversing heart and vascular disease.

You have more power over this killer than you realize. Heart disease is a problem we bring upon ourselves. We're not helpless,

Ask the Holistic Heart Doc:
How do I know which prescriptions to try first?

The answer to that question is this: It depends. In Part Two of this book, I've organized the chapters in order from the most pressing and immediate to things you can tackle later. So if you want to make a lot of impact early, incorporate as many of the prescriptions from Chapter 6 as you can. Then tackle Chapter 7. Then Chapter 8. You get the idea.

Within each chapter, however, you'll find the prescriptions ordered by their ease of implementation. So if you worry about biting off more than you can chew (pun intended), go easy on yourself. Tackle the and we don't necessarily need state-of-the-art medicine to do anything about it.

You can prevent and reverse blockages. You really can, and you can do it no matter what kind of health insurance you have.

It is my hope that the time you spend reading this book will help you to avoid ever having to fill expensive prescriptions for life-saving medications, as well as a trip to an emergency room, catheter lab, or surgical suite. It is possible to ward off heart disease and the limitations it imposes on your life. The secret is in your hands.

Please join me for this lecture, the one I wanted to give but didn't have enough time to deliver.

It is starting now, and it just might save your life.

prescriptions in the order they are presented. That way, you'll be able to slowly wade into the heart-healthy waters.

Or, you can break it down even more by making your first goal a simple one: Read this book from cover to cover. As you do so, make a list of prescriptions that seem feasible to you, and tackle those prescriptions first. As you experience some success, try a few that seem a little more difficult, and so on.

Ideally, for a healthy heart and a long and joyful life, you'll want to incorporate as many prescriptions as possible. But whether you start with the most effective remedies or the easiest to implement makes little difference. One way or another, you'll eventually end up in good health.

Chapter 2

It Takes a Body to Beat a Heart

When Gwen began feeling pain on the left side of her chest, she went straight to the emergency room. That's where the 66-year-old woman learned that one of the arteries leading to her heart was 80 percent blocked. Another crucial heart artery was 90 percent clogged.

Gwen underwent bypass surgery for advanced heart blockages.

Betty, her identical twin, had never experienced chest pain or shortness of breath. Still, she was concerned. The two shared the same DNA. If Gwen had heart disease, wouldn't Betty have it, too?

Betty made an appointment with her health care provider. Health care professionals wired Betty with sensors. Then she got on a treadmill and started walking. After just three minutes, her health care provider asked her to step off the treadmill; he didn't like what he was seeing on the readout.

Sure enough, the results of another test revealed that two of the arteries leading to Betty's heart were between 70 and 80 percent blocked.

She underwent bypass surgery, too.[8]

YOUR NOT-SO-GENETIC INHERITANCE

The story of Betty and Gwen is a real one. I've changed their names, but otherwise all of the details are the same. I read about them in a case study about identical twins and how their genetics do or do not predict their health outcomes. Stories like theirs saturate medical literature. On the surface, they make it seem as if the progression of heart disease is predetermined. Inherit a set of heart disease–causing genes—as Betty and Gwen seem to have done—and, voila, you eventually develop heart disease. Case closed.

Or is it?

As it turns out, while our genetic inheritance certainly plays a role, it doesn't play as much of a role as many scientists once thought. What large, multiyear studies of identical twins tell us is this: The Bettys and Gwens of the world are actually quite rare. More often than not, identical twins don't suffer the same fate. One twin might get breast cancer while the other develops diabetes. Another might live to age 90 while her sister dies years earlier. Yet another might undergo bypass surgery at age 50 while his twin brother never has a need to fill a prescription for a cholesterol-lowering medication.

Professor Tim Spector, head of twin research at King's College in London, has studied thousands of twins for many decades. He's mapped their genomes and tracked their health outcomes. According to his research, twins rarely die from the same disease, and this is true even when they are identical. Yes, even if twins share the same DNA, the code of instructions for our bodies, if one of them develops heart disease, there's only a 30 percent chance the remaining twin will get it, too. Spector has even written a book about this phenomenon called *Identically Different*.

How can this possibly be? As it turns out, the human body is much more complex than previously thought. Some things, such as nearsightedness and acne, are much more inheritable than others, such as blood pressure. Also, very few single genes cause any

Heart Disease 101

Heart disease isn't just one health problem. It's actually made up of different issues that work either in isolation or together to damage your heart. It can include:

Blood cholesterol. When certain types of blood cholesterol are abnormal, the main arteries leading to the heart are more likely to become clogged.

High blood pressure. When your arteries become stiff and/or narrowed, the pressure inside them builds, which causes blood flow to become more turbulent. End result: The lining of the arteries is more likely to become damaged.

Heart attack. This happens when a blood clot blocks the flow of blood through one or more of the blood vessels that feed the heart muscle. Interrupted blood flow to the heart can damage or destroy a part of the heart muscle.

Stroke. This is just like a heart attack, but it happens inside the brain. Arteries leading to the brain are narrowed or blocked and too little blood reaches it, causing some of your brain cells to die.

Heart failure. Heart failure occurs when a heart can't pump enough blood to meet a body's needs. This often happens after a heart attack, when the heart is too damaged to pump normally.

one disease. Health or lack of it develops as a result of *hundreds* of different genes, all influencing one another to either trigger disease or stop it from developing. ***Most important: Your lifestyle can switch those genes on and off.*** Do healthy things—exercise, eat right, meditate—and you switch on the genes that promote good health. Do unhealthy things—smoke, eat foods laced with pesticides, sit a lot—and you switch off those healthy genes and switch on the unhealthy ones.

This is just one example of how the health of your heart is affected by factors that, on the surface, have very little to do with your heart at all. Indeed, for a healthy heart, you need more than just healthy blood vessels. You also need healthy DNA and healthy cells and healthy proteins and tissues and organs and even healthy microbes inside your GI tract. As it turns out, it takes an entire body to keep your heart beating. Let's take a closer look at how it all works.

THE WHOLE HEART DISEASE PICTURE

For many years, we thought that the heart was nothing more than a mechanical pump that took oxygen-depleted blood and sent it to the lungs. There, in the lungs, cells became infused with oxygen, turning the blood red. Then the blood flowed back into the left side of the heart and throughout the rest of the body.

Like most pumps, it was thought that the fist-sized heart would keep working as long as it had an uninterrupted supply of fuel. Cut off the source of fuel (in this case, blood) and the pump malfunctioned or stopped working altogether. If you kept the blood flowing by making sure the arteries didn't get clogged, everything would work just fine.

Or so it was thought.

We now know that the heart is much more than a pump. It's really a miniature brain—complete with its own set of neurons— and emits its own hormones and even an electrical field. As a result, for us to experience optimal health, we need much more than merely a healthy pump. We need healthy neurons within that pump. We also need healthy nerves that connect it to the brain and other parts of the body. Similarly, that pump needs healthy cells, so it can contract and relax with enough force to send blood all the way from the top of the head down to the pinky toe and then bring oxygen-depleted blood all the way back up to the lungs. And those cells need nutrients and co-factors . . . the cycle goes on and on and on.

For optimum heart health, it's important to make sure every

cell in your body functions optimally. Only caring for your heart and blood vessels—and ignoring the health of the rest of your body—is like only monitoring the spark plugs of your car, but never taking steps to change the oil or do any other upkeep. Eventually, the engine stops running.

Cardiologists should care for more than just the cardiovascular system, just as pulmonologists should care for more than just the lungs and neurologists for more than just the brain. Sure, we specialize in these organs and systems, but if we ignore the health of the rest of the body, our patients will never experience true, good health. That's why I promote holistic health, viewing the body holistically and as a web of interconnected organs, tissues, and cells, all of which are influenced by nearly everything you think, say, and do. Your genes play a role. So do the foods you eat, as does every other part of your lifestyle. Let's take a closer look at this amazing system, and how all of the parts work holistically in tandem to ensure good health—or bad.

IT TAKES BLOOD VESSELS TO BEAT A HEART

Arteries carry oxygen-rich red blood away from the heart and veins carry spent blue blood toward it. Think of arteries like the tracks that carry trains to destinations that need their cargo. Think of veins like the tracks that carry the empty trains back to the depot, so they can be reloaded.

No matter where a blood vessel exists in your body—whether it carries blood to the brain, to your heart, or to your sex organs—its vitality matters. Diseased blood vessels to the genitals, for example, lead to erectile dysfunction. Diseased blood vessels to the eyes can cause vision problems and blindness.

And you can probably guess what diseased blood vessels leading to the heart cause: heart attacks. Your heart arteries are called *coronary arteries* because they make a crown or corona around the heart muscle, and they are among the most important arteries to keep clear, for obvious reasons.

There are three, equal-sized coronary arteries surrounding the heart, lying on top of the muscle within a small amount of fat to cushion them. If you could take a trip with me to a cadaver lab and watch me as I sliced one open, you'd be able to see just how thin and delicate a healthy blood vessel is. The inner area of an artery, called the lumen, behaves somewhat like the inside of a pipe. It allows blood to travel to the hungry heart muscle to supply oxygen and nutrients. Arteries also have a single layer of super cells called the endothelium that line the inside of the lumen. These cells keep the artery resistant to injury and clotting. When they are healthy, they also allow the artery to relax (or dilate) to provide more blood flow when needed. More than 400 years ago Thomas Sydenham said, "A man is as old as his arteries." In reality, you are as old as the endothelial lining of your arteries.

When your lifestyle is not healthy, the endothelium deteriorates. When that happens, your arteries start to clog with plaque (irritated segments of the arteries that are full of cholesterol, calcium, scar tissue, and cells) and clots can more easily form. They can clog 30, 50, 70 percent or even more without giving you a single symptom of disease.

We once thought that arteries narrowed in a straightforward, predictable way: You consume foods rich in fat and cholesterol, particularly the saturated fats found in meat, eggs, and dairy. The fat and cholesterol enter through the intestine and travel into the bloodstream; the cholesterol travels in small packages called lipoproteins. If too much cholesterol comes in over time, the arteries narrow, cutting off the blood supply to the heart.

We now know that this process is much more complex. Not all cholesterol is created equal. The two major kinds of lipoproteins are low-density lipoprotein (LDL) cholesterol and high-density lipoprotein (HDL) cholesterol. LDL cholesterol is sometimes called "bad" cholesterol. This is because it carries cholesterol to tissues, including your heart arteries. HDL cholesterol is sometimes called "good" cholesterol because it acts like a vacuum cleaner for the arteries, helping to sop up bad cholesterol and take it to the liver for disposal.

But it's even more complex than that. Not all LDL or HDL cholesterol is created equal, either. Two people can both have an LDL cholesterol level of 100 mg/dl (milligrams per deciliter of blood) and be told by their health care provider that things look good but, in reality, be at very different risks for heart attacks. One of them might be at high risk, and, if he doesn't get his diet and lifestyle under control, he might think about picking out a casket. The other might be at very low risk. How can this be?

We now know that someone with an LDL cholesterol level of 100 mg/dl may really have many LDL particles with only a small amount of cholesterol in each one. This is similar to a stretch of highway with 100 passengers. If they are driving 10 to a minivan, then there are only 10 large vehicles on the road and it is not too congested. If all 100 are riding in individual small cars, think of the congestion on the road now. That is how large and small LDL appears in arteries. Lots of LDL particles clog up the artery highway.

If you allow me to change up the metaphor, those 100 LDL riders in small cars can also be hard and dense, like a golf ball. Alternatively, the minivan type of LDLs can be large, soft, and fluffy, more like a sponge ball. I ask my patients which is easier to break a screened-in window with: a small golf ball or a larger sponge ball? Well, it turns out the walls of arteries are similar to window screens, and small, dense LDL particles (golf balls) do a lot of damage to those screens.

So let's get back to those two people with an LDL level of 100 mg/dl. Their heart disease risk can vary wildly because it's possible that they have widely different particle numbers and sizes. One may have well under 1,000 LDL particles in a blood sample, and the size of the LDL may be large like sponge balls, so their risk for hardening of arteries is low. The second person might have a particle number of over 2,000 and be loaded with small "golf balls" that are knocking into and entering arteries to cause plaques.

Just as some LDLs are more harmful than others, some HDLs are also more helpful than others. We used to think that HDL was such an easy particle in the blood to appreciate. It was the particle wearing a white hat with a big H on it for "Happy." All it did was stream through the blood vessels and perform RCT *(reverse cholesterol transport)*. RCT is a miracle. The HDL particle removes cholesterol from plaques and decreases the severity of blockages, much like a vacuum cleaner for the arteries. So the higher your HDL, the lower your chances of heart disease, right?

Well, that's what many of us thought until somewhat recently.

But it's not true. HDL seems to be closely tied to the immune system. Evidence suggests that someone with an extremely high HDL might not be healthy at all. Rather, those HDLs might be elevated because the immune system is fighting off an infection somewhere in the body. Those high levels of HDLs might, in reality, be a sign that someone has gum disease, a urinary tract infection, or even colitis. Low-grade reactions to dairy, corn, soy, or wheat gluten might spike HDLs as well. Furthermore, HDL particles have recently been shown to promote atherosclerosis in some circumstances!

In addition, HDL has to be functional to vacuum effectively. In the huge and complex HDL molecule is an enzyme called *paraoxanase* that works to improve arterial health. Although we have no way to measure it with an office test, we know that this enzyme must be functioning in order for HDL to work its magic, and, in some people, toxins from food, water, or even self-care products have poisoned it, stopping the enzyme from working effectively.

Now, here's where things get even more complicated. Equally important as the number, type, and size of cholesterol inside your arteries is the health of the arteries themselves. Healthy arteries can withstand a lot more abuse than unhealthy arteries. Many other factors are also important, including:

How much oxygen is stressing your cells. Every breath transfers oxygen to tissues throughout the body, and oxygen is to our bodies what water is to a houseplant. Too little of it and you die; just the right amount and you thrive. Too much and cells throughout your body undergo stress, just like a plant drowning in too much of a good thing.

Oxidative stress damages organs, tissues, cells, DNA, proteins, cell membranes, and even cholesterol molecules. LDL cholesterol has little ability to clog the arteries on its own. When it is damaged by oxygen, however, the oxidized LDL is recognized as foreign by the lining of the arteries, and this causes plaques to build up.

A certain amount of oxidative stress is inevitable. You can't stop breathing, for instance, but you can take steps to ensure that your body undergoes no more oxidative stress than needed. You can also keep your body's natural oxidation control team on high alert, ready to prevent and repair oxidative damage as it takes place. This oxidation control team consists of enzymes called catalase, superoxide dismutase, and glutathione peroxidase. That's quite a mouthful, but these enzymes prevent our tissues, cells, and DNA from getting damaged when exposed to oxygen. Smoking, processed foods laden with chemicals and toxins, heavy metals like mercury in fish, and inadequate sleep, among many other things, can also harm or hinder these enzymes, allowing oxidation to operate unchecked. Certain nutrients, on the other hand, support these enzymes. *Limit the harmful stress nutrients and maximize the right ones, and LDL cholesterol is rendered less harmful.*

How much sugar is floating around in your bloodstream. Glycation is what happens when the glucose (sugar) in your blood coats proteins and important lipids. This process can affect any protein or lipid in the body, including cholesterol. When LDL cholesterol becomes glycated, it's more likely to irritate arteries and build up as plaque.

The process of glycation can go a step further to create dangerous particles called advanced glycation end products (AGEs).

These extremely damaging substances accelerate aging through-out the body, speeding the progression of everything from heart disease to diabetes to wrinkles to stroke. You can fight wrinkles and heart disease at the same time with the prescriptions in this book!

There are two sources of AGEs: internal and external. First, let's look at internal sources of AGEs. When our blood sugar rises too high for too long (usually from consuming too many sugary, starchy, processed foods), proteins and lipids become coated by the elevated sugars. Hemoglobin inside red blood cells can also be coated by elevated blood sugars and hemoglobin A1C (HgbA1C) is a common test that measures this process in the bloodstream. The second source of AGEs comes from our food. Specifically, the way food is prepared has a huge effect on the quantity of AGEs that then get absorbed into our bodies. You'll learn more about this in Chapter 7.

Whether your immune system is on high alert. When a mos-quito lands on your back and dines on some of your blood, your body responds to the bite with pain, warmth, redness, and swell-ing. That's an immune reaction called *inflammation*. Remember this word because I'm pretty sure it's in every chapter of this book. If you like science, here's how it works. Immune cells survey their environment all the time with detectors on their surfaces that act much like radar. These detectors are called *pattern recognition receptors (PRRs)*. If a PRR detects something that has a foreign structure—a *pathogen-associated molecular pattern (PAMP)*—it will ring the fire alarm. Chemicals then cause blood vessels to dilate (creating redness, warmth, and swelling); others increase the sensitivity to pain, and the next thing you know, your ankle or finger is a hot, red, sore mess. Histamine is one of the chemi-cals involved in this process. It causes arteries to expand and leak fluid (such as the runny nose you get when your body is invaded by a cold virus; thus, you need to take an antihistamine pill to dry up your nose). Other chemicals called interleukins, such as IL-8, come from macrophages (blood cells that gobble up bacteria and regulate immunity) and bring their best friends: white blood cells. The white cells arrive to fight for your recovery because chemical attractants—sort of a white blood cell perfume—are released. Tumor necrosis factor alpha (TNF-alpha) also is released from macrophage cells, and may produce fever and loss of appetite. Nitric oxide is a gas released by the inner lining of blood cells and can be dumped out to increase blood flow when an injury occurs.

When I explain inflammation to patients, I point out that the middle of the word is "flame" and that it comes from the Latin "I ignite." Think of a fire going off in your body, particularly in your arteries. That's because, while acute inflammation like that caused by a mosquito bite protects our health, chronic inflammation is a different story. Imagine it this way. The mosquito is long dead, but your body keeps pumping chemicals and extra blood flow for months and the bump never goes away.

A diverse group of medical illnesses are believed to be caused in part by chronic inflammation. These include asthma, acne, celiac disease, rheumatoid arthritis, and even atherosclerosis of heart arteries. Chronic inflammation is also thought to block cells from recognizing the hormone insulin. When cells become insulin resistant, blood sugar rises. It also might keep brain cells from listening to the hormone leptin, causing your appetite switch to malfunction and allowing you to hungrily eat many more calories than your body needs.

In many ways, inflammation is a "Goldilocks" process; you don't want too much or too little, but just the right amount. Many of the prescriptions in this book are designed to help you keep pro- and anti-inflammatory reactions in the "Goldilocks" just right position.

IT TAKES DNA TO BEAT A HEART

You may or may not remember from high school biology that deoxyribonucleic acid (DNA) is a molecule that contains a set of instructions. It clusters together within the body to create chromosomes, and it exists in every single cell.

Depending on the DNA in your cells, you might be more or less susceptible to heart disease. For instance, because of your DNA, it might be harder for you to keep a lid on your blood cholesterol, blood sugar, or blood pressure than it is for someone else.[9]

The good news, as I mentioned earlier, is that you are not trapped by your genetic inheritance. Your cells might contain genes for heart disease, Alzheimer's, or breast cancer, but those genes can lie dormant for years and even for a lifetime. *Genes must get switched on in order to function, and that's why a heart-healthy lifestyle is so important.* If you follow the whole heart prescriptions in this book, you can prevent any heart disease genes from turning on and thus escape your family history while at the same time lowering your risk of obesity, Alzheimer's disease, cancer, and diabetes. Here's more: Even if an unhealthy lifestyle has already activated these disease-causing genes, you can flip them back off.

In this way nurture (your lifestyle) acts on nature (your genes) to affect your future. Scientists call this process *epigenetics.*

This first came to light when researchers were studying the health of identical twins, as I mentioned earlier. These types of twins share the same genetic code, but when researchers tracked their health, they found that the twins had different rates of chronic diseases. How could this be if their genes determined their fate? Epigenetic modification of the genes is part of the answer. Your body has methods to switch genes on and off and you can control this process by adopting a heart-healthy lifestyle.

The proof comes from work done in the laboratory of Dean Ornish, MD, a cardiologist famous for showing that the progression of heart disease can be reversed by a low-stress lifestyle, plant-based foods, exercise, and social support. Early in Ornish's career, he gathered 48 patients who had been diagnosed with artery blockages, and he taught 28 of them how to follow a low-fat, vegetarian diet. He told them to quit smoking, encouraged moderate exercise, and taught them stress management techniques. The other 20 patients received usual care. At the end of a year, 82 percent of the patients in the diet and lifestyle group had smaller and fewer blockages. The blood flow to their hearts had also improved. The usual care group, on the other hand, had bigger blockages and less blood flow. Ornish kept track of these patients for many years, and the trend has continued.[10] Nurture trumped nature in this most sophisticated of studies.

More recently, Ornish showed that three months of a diet rich in plant-based foods containing less than 10 percent fat, moderate exercise, social support, and mind/body stress reduction activities like yoga not only helped study participants drop weight, blood pressure, and blood cholesterol, but also helped them turn on the genes for good health and turn off the genes for poor health. This result came about in just three months![11] He worked with a Nobel Prize–winning scientist, Elizabeth Blackburn, PhD, and the implications of turning your genes into health-producing machines in a short time frame are revolutionary.

The message emerging on epigenetics is both clear and hopeful. If you give your genes the right raw materials, they will help you to keep blood pressure, cholesterol, and other heart disease risk factors in check. I've incorporated Dr. Ornish's findings, along with other research about what works to turn on the right genes, into my whole heart prescriptions. This approach has allowed me to help patients heal even the worst blockages—even ones so advanced that they were starving the heart and leading to chest pain.

One way to feed your genes the raw materials they need is to make sure you methylate optimally. No, I'm not making that word up! A methyl group is a carbon atom with three hydrogen atoms. All you need to understand is that the body adds or removes methyl groups in order to switch DNA molecules on or off.

Warning: more science. One step of the methylation cycle that is in every cell in our bodies involves the enzyme MTHFR (methyltetrahydrofolate reductase). About 40 percent of the population carries a gene or two that slows functioning of the MTHFR enzyme. I carry one of these defective genes. If a blood test reveals that you carry one or two of these bad gene copies, it's very important that you feed your MTHFR enzymes the fuel they need to operate optimally. What is that fuel? It's the same B vitamins found in most dark leafy greens: folate and B_6. You also need plenty of B_{12}. It's best to take these as a supplement along with healthy foods because you need them in a special form if your MTHFR gene is defective. This form is called methylated vitamins. Many companies make methyl B_{12} (methylcobalamin), methyl folate (MTHF), and B_6 as pyridoxal phosphate along with TMG (betaine, which is used to help the other vitamins work optimally). Healthy methylation not only improves endothelial artery function but may have profound effects on lowering the risk of autism, cancer, and other diseases.

IT TAKES A THYROID GLAND TO BEAT A HEART

The thyroid gland, which sits about a foot above the heart by the Adam's apple, can have a profound influence on cardiovascular health. About two percent of people have an overactive thyroid (hyperthyroidism). Thyroid hormones like T4 and T3 increase the activity of the heart and may result in an elevated heart rate, arrhythmias like atrial fibrillation, hypertension, and even a weakness of the heart muscle called a cardiomyopathy. Fatigue, weight loss, shortness of breath, palpitations, and an elevated temperature may result.

Another five percent have an underactive thyroid (hypothyroidism). This produces fatigue, weight gain, constipation, slowed heart rates, low temperatures, and elevations in blood sugar and cholesterol levels. Hypothyroidism is associated with accelerated hardening of the arteries as well as elevated levels of homocysteine (an amino acid important in artery health that is produced by the methylation cycle I just told you about), high-sensitivity C-reactive protein (a marker of vessel inflammation), and blood clotting.

The bottom line is this: To have a healthy heart, you also need a healthy thyroid.

IT TAKES AN ADRENAL GLAND TO BEAT A HEART

The stress hormone cortisol is made by the adrenal glands, located above the kidneys, and it's the only hormone that increases with age.

Cortisol is at its highest levels in the morning and falls to lower levels by night, only to repeat the cycle again in a daily pattern. Unfortunately, modern life is often characterized by chronic stress, poor sleep, changing work shifts, and poor nutrition, which can result in elevated cortisol levels throughout much of the day.

Part of the fight-or-flight response, excess cortisol drives up blood sugars, cholesterol, and blood pressure. It also impairs thyroid function and renders cells and tissues resistant to the hormone insulin, which can raise blood sugar and worsen inflammation. Altered immune function and accelerated osteoporosis also frequently result.

If cortisol remains elevated for a long period of time, the adrenal gland can actually wear out. Called adrenal fatigue or burnout, this condition is characterized by lower than normal cortisol levels. Fatigue, along with insomnia, diminished sexual interest, and low blood pressure may manifest. Many athletes who train for repeated endurance events develop adrenal fatigue.

IT TAKES SEX ORGANS TO BEAT A HEART

Cardiovascular disease develops an average of 10 years earlier in men than in women. Why? The culprit might be a life transition known as male menopause. Although not as publicized or dramatic as female menopause, men do have their own change. Testosterone levels begin to decline about one percent each year, beginning at age 30.

Studies have found lower levels of testosterone in men with coronary artery disease than in those without heart issues, and testosterone replacement therapy may lower cholesterol and blood pressure, and improve arterial stiffness, insulin sensitivity, and blood glucose levels. Studies have shown relief of angina pectoris (chest pain) with testosterone replacement therapy.

Like men, women's risk of heart disease rises sharply after menopause, and levels of protective female hormones drop. But, for women, hormone replacement therapy is more complicated. Let's turn the clock back to 2002. Back then there was a general feeling that menopause should be treated with replacement hormones to boost falling estrogen and progesterone levels. The rationale was that hormone replacement therapy (HRT) could relieve symptoms while also helping to boost memory, strengthen bones, and prevent the rise in heart disease that occurs in postmenopausal women.

In 2002 the Women's Health Initiative evaluated the results of using HRT in more than 16,000 women. Researchers halted the estrogen/progestin arm of the study early because an increased risk of heart disease and breast cancer was found. The researchers concluded that HRT should not be used for the primary prevention of coronary artery heart disease. Two years later another part of the study, using only estrogen replacement, was terminated due to an increase in stroke.

Is this an open and shut case? No. New research shows that starting HRT earlier, at the onset of menopause, does not cause the same harmful health effects as starting it later.[12] It's also possible that HRT raised heart risk because of the way it was manufactured. The HRT used in the study (and by most patients at that time) was not identical to the chemicals found in a woman's body. The estrogen was created from a concentrated source of female horse urine (conjugated equine estrogen) and the progesterone component came from a synthetic progestin, not the natural progesterone chemical found in the blood of healthy women.

It's possible that hormones that more closely resemble true estrogen and progesterone could still benefit women's heart health and overall health, too. Smaller studies using individualized doses of natural HRT—often called bioidentical hormones—used topically are promising, showing that bioidentical hormones may not cause the harmful side effects that synthetic ones do.[13]

Yes, bioidentical hormones are not yet a proven therapy, but I've seen how dramatically a patient's health is transformed once she starts using these hormones. If you are a woman with symptoms of perimenopause or wishing to explore the risks and benefits of HRT in general, find a practitioner experienced in these therapies and determine if HRT of any kind is a good option for you. Avoid oral forms of estrogen and testosterone, as they quickly degrade once they pass through the liver, possibly producing harmful compounds. Explore patches and compounded creams.

IT TAKES A GUT TO BEAT A HEART

If someone asked you what you were made of, I'm guessing that you probably wouldn't answer with, "Bacteria! I'm made of bacteria!"

But, if you did, you'd be right on the money.

We contain 10 times more microbial cells inside our bodies than human ones, and, whether any of us like to admit it, we share about 37 percent of our genes with these little bugs.

Our guts, for instance, are lined with trillions of bacteria that help us digest our food, make vitamins, build and maintain the intestinal wall, and even program the immune system. If we have the right mix of bacteria, they can switch on the good DNA and turn off the bad DNA. They also emit chemicals that promote good health and good mood, and crowd out the organisms that cause bad health.

On the other hand, if our intestines are chock-full of the wrong types of bacteria, these tiny beings can break down and convert certain food nutrients into toxins that irritate the linings of the arteries and cause plaque to build up.

As a result, the right mix of bacteria can reduce our risk of developing everything from obesity to diabetes to high blood pressure to heart disease to depression. We inherit some of our gut flora from our mothers. Babies born vaginally end up with a healthier mix of bacteria in their GI tracts throughout life than babies delivered by C-section![14] We pick up other bacteria over time, for better or worse. As it turns out, our modern lifestyles might be tipping the gut flora balance toward the "worse" and away from the "better." Overuse of antibiotics, for instance, serves as an atomic bomb for populations of good bacteria. And certain animal fats and sugar-rich processed foods tend to nourish harmful bacteria and starve the good guys, setting the stage for heart disease, obesity, and diabetes.

IT TAKES ELECTRICITY TO BEAT A HEART

A few years ago Dr. Mehmet Oz was quoted on *The Oprah Winfrey Show* as saying that "energy medicine is the future of all medicine."

What was he talking about?

Your heart cannot beat without energy. In fact, without energy, you would be dead. Electrical currents cross every cell membrane and mitochondrial membrane (the powerhouses inside every cell that generate ATP energy like a generator) as sodium and potassium are shuttled back and forth. It's electrical surges (called action potentials) that cause every cell to contract and relax. When heart cells contract in unison, your heart pumps blood efficiently. When they relax in unison, your heart relaxes with them and easily fills back up with blood.

Pacemakers and defibrillators work based on this principle, pacing or shocking the heart out of lethal rhythms. These surges of energy can keep the heart beating in an organized and regular manner. Years ago I had a patient who would grab on to the electrical posts of his truck battery when his heart went out of rhythm. It's not necessarily a tactic I would ever recommend, but it worked many times for him. I gave him an A for ingenuity, but advised him to stop this unpredictable and unconventional practice. Instead, I recommended a controlled electrical cardioversion in the hospital to fix the problem that was causing his heart to beat erratically.

The human body is really just one large battery, one that emits a field of energy that can be measured up to several feet away. In fact, we can interact with the energy fields of other living creatures around us.

If we interact with energy sources that differ greatly from the energy of our hearts—for instance with the energy emitted by cell phones and microwaves—this theoretically could disturb the heart's natural rhythm, especially in susceptible people. On the other hand, if we closely interact with positive energy sources (such as the energy emitted by other living beings and the Earth itself), we can enhance our heart health. When scientists at the nonprofit Institute for HeartMath monitored the heart and brain rhythms of couples, mothers, and infants, and even people with their pets, they found that their heart rhythms synchronize and beat in unison when they are in close proximity.[15] This is called coherence and is a powerful tool that can be used to improve heart health. This might all sound fairly New Age and far out, but considering nearly everyone now walks around with a cell phone in their breast pocket, it has taken on new importance.

THE SECRET TO WHOLE BODY HEART HEALTH

By now I hope I've convinced you. To prevent everyone's number one killer, you must do more than protect your heart and the arteries that carry blood to it. You want to ensure the health of every organ, tissue, cell, and molecule inside your body.

This leads me directly into the point I will make in the next chapter. No one drug and no one office procedure could ever protect every single cell in your body. So for optimal heart protection, you want to make the most of a heart-healthy lifestyle—doing everything in your power to ensure the beat goes on for days, weeks, months, years, and decades to come.

The prescriptions in this book will show you how.

Chapter 3

Why Drugs and Surgery Aren't the Answer

During the first half of the 1990s, the United States and several other countries refused to do trade with communist Cuba. During what is now known as "the special period," Cubans were isolated from the rest of the world, and citizens were forced to find ways to go without imported luxuries like cars and even many foods.

We think of Cuba as a country full of 1950s-style cars. In reality, most people got around during those years with bicycles or by walking. When they had to haul a heavy load, they used a donkey.

Many countries lifted these restrictions in 1995, and Cubans began returning to a modern, sedentary, calorie-rich life.

This was a boon for health scientists, especially because the Cuban government was fastidious about record keeping. When a team of researchers from Cuba, Spain, and the United States wanted to see how "the special period" affected the health of the average Cuban, they had plenty of records to work with.

After they crunched the numbers, the lesson was both startling and very clear. Between 1991 and 1995, when most Cubans used their own two feet for transportation, the average Cuban dropped nine pounds. As a result, rates of diabetes and deaths from heart attacks and strokes plummeted. In comparison, between 1995 and 2010, after most of the restrictions were lifted, the average Cuban gained 19 pounds, and rates of heart disease and diabetes ballooned right along with those expanding midsections.

If a similar "special period" took place in the United States, Canada, or any other industrialized country, it would slash death rates from heart disease by a third and diabetes by half, experts predict.[16] A similar example: In New York, where many people need to walk (and usually walk briskly!) to get to where they're going, heart health is better on average than in other major cities.

As this research shows, both the prevention and cure for heart disease are very simple. Indeed, the most potent medicines and treatments for heart disease are found not in a physician's office, pharmacy, or hospital. They have less to do with technology, innovation, or even medications and much more to do with what you think, do, and eat.

That's why most of the prescriptions you'll find throughout the pages of this book will cost you nothing to implement. No matter where you live, you will be able to find them, afford them, and use them. I'm guessing at least a few of those remedies are actually already inside your house.

Are there any vegetables in your refrigerator? Is there a pair of walking shoes anywhere in a closet? How about some sunshine? Got any of that? Can you breathe slowly and deeply?

These natural prescriptions and many more serve as powerful weapons that halt inflammation, protect your cells from oxidation, and keep all of the tissues in your body young, vibrant, and healthy.

So why are so many people ignoring these easily available heart protectors and instead opting for prescription drugs and even surgery? I'll tell you why: false security. People erroneously think that prescription medications and office procedures are all they need to fend off the number one killer of men and women.

This couldn't be further from the truth.

Please don't misunderstand me. I'm not saying that you will never need a cholesterol-lowering medication or bypass surgery.

For some people prescription medications and surgical options can be lifesaving. But the sad fact of the matter is this: In most cases, their use could have been prevented with simple lifestyle changes. And those lifestyle changes are, by far, the better option.

Let's take a look at why.

WHY WONDER DRUGS AREN'T ALWAYS WONDERFUL

Every chance I get—even if I'm just chatting with the person standing near me at a checkout counter—I recommend consuming a whole food, plant-based diet. I also ask all my patients to read books and videos about heart-healthy lifestyles, because taking a prescription heart drug without changing your lifestyle is like waiting until after you've slipped off the edge of a waterfall to call 911 without bothering to put up a protective fence to prevent its happening in the first place. The lifestyle changes described in this book are that fence. They will stop you from falling into a heart attack, stroke, or even a funeral home.

A body-wide disease requires a body-wide treatment. Prescription medications, heart stents, and bypass operations do not treat a whole body problem. For optimal heart protection, you want your body to be in optimal health—and that's something no procedure can do for you.

Statins

Have you ever heard the words "3-hydroxy-3-methylglutaryl coenzyme A reductase inhibitor"? That's the long-winded chemical name for a statin, a type of cholesterol-lowering medication. The first one, lovastatin, obtained approval from the U.S. Food and Drug Administration in 1987. Since then others have hit the market: atorvastatin (Lipitor), simvastatin (Zocor), pravastatin

(Pravachol), rosuvastatin (Crestor), and others. Now they are the most prescribed drugs in the world, with sales in the billions of dollars.

According to the National Center for Health Statistics, in the United States 18 percent of men older than 45 now take statins, up from just 15 percent in the late 1990s, and three percent in the late 1980s and early 1990s.[17] In Canada, 30 million statin prescriptions are filled each year, and $2 billion spent in the process.

Statins work by inhibiting the activity of an enzyme called 3-hydroxy-3-methylglutaryl-coenyzme A reductase (thus the reason for their long chemical name). When this enzyme is blocked, the liver makes less cholesterol. Consequently blood levels of cholesterol fall. They also suppress inflammation and enhance the function of the inner lining of arteries called the endothelium.

And they work. When I put patients on the maximum dose for a statin, their total and LDL cholesterol drops by 50 percent or more. That's an impressive result, one that may lead to improved arterial health, especially in people whose cholesterol levels start out above 300 mg/dl. For every 1-millimole-per-liter reduction in blood cholesterol levels, statins reduce the risk of a heart attack in high-risk patients by 10 to 20 percent.

Since the introduction of these drugs, death rates from heart disease have been cut in half.[18] That's a dramatic outcome, one that I don't argue with one bit. Statins are so powerfully effective at lowering cholesterol that some enthusiastic cardiologists say, "they should be put into the drinking water." Others believe in statins so much, they argue they should be available over-the-counter, so more people can take them, even young people with no existing evidence of heart disease. An eminent professor of cardiology has boldly said that the only side effect of statins is a reduction in heart attack and strokes.

So why aren't they the answer for all? Why can't we all just take a statin with our Big Mac and call it a day? Let me count the ways. Statins are not the answer, because:

They treat only a small part of a body-wide problem. Remember what I told you in Chapter 2: It takes an entire body to beat a heart, and cholesterol levels are only one small piece of the larger heart disease puzzle. Case in point: Some people with cholesterol levels above 300 mg/dl have fairly clear arteries whereas others with levels below 170 end up having heart attacks. If cholesterol were the only cause of heart disease, that just wouldn't be the case. Statins don't address sleep, stress, diet, exercise, or many other factors that affect arteries.

They mask the true problem. In many cases the real problem may not be just high cholesterol, but the lifestyle factors that drive it upwards. Using a drug without solving the lifestyle problem is a lot like turning over a stained couch cushion: You don't remove the stain; you merely hide it.

They pose many undesirable side effects. Soon after starting statin therapy, quite a few patients tell me that their memory becomes a problem and they ask to come off the medication. This is a problem that fortunately reverses itself when they stop taking the medicines. Up to 60 percent of patients taking the highest doses of statin medications report fatigue, muscle weakness, and joint pain.[19] This side effect might stem from alterations in muscle metabolism and particularly the function of mitochondria. Mitochondria are the powerhouses of all cells, particularly muscle and heart muscle cells. In volunteers taking statins, enzyme levels related to mitochondrial health fall, which is why some health professionals have nicknamed them "mitochondrial poisons."[20]

They raise risk for other serious diseases. One of the side effects of statins? They may raise blood sugar, and postmenopausal women who take statins are 48 percent more likely to end up with diabetes.[21] It's thought that the drugs reduce the action of glucose receptors on cells, keeping blood sugar high. It is ironic and unfortunate that a medicine used to reduce heart disease might hasten the onset of diabetes and the accelerated vessel damage associated with that condition. This is a serious concern. Another recent study that looked at the medical records of two million patients in the United States, Canada, and Britain linked statin use with a slightly increased risk of kidney injury.[22]

They block the health benefits of other just-as-healthy treatments. Exercise is one of the most potent heart disease fighters around, and any improvement in fitness has been shown to drop your risk of death by 50 percent.[23] That's a huge benefit. Statins, unfortunately, have recently been shown to hinder the effectiveness of exercise. When researchers compared new exercisers who were taking statins to those who weren't, the new exercisers not taking statins boosted their fitness by 10 percent whereas the statin group only boosted fitness by a mere one percent.[24]

They lower one risk factor for heart disease by raising another. As statins block the production of cholesterol, they also block the production of other metabolites including Coenzyme Q10 (CoQ10), the main antioxidant in cells and an essential factor in producing energy in cells. Although I admit that the data supporting the routine use of CoQ10 supplements in all patients taking statins is not yet strong enough to win a debate, I favor the routine use of this strong antioxidant with a high safety margin for all of my patients who must take a statin to lower their cholesterol level.

Some are sold for a Cadillac price when a Kia is available. Researchers at the University Medical Center in Rotterdam looked at data from the Framingham Heart Study and the Framingham Offspring Study, both of which tracked the lifestyle habits and health outcomes of thousands of people over many years. They used that data to measure the cost effectiveness of four different interventions: smoking cessation, blood pressure medicines, aspirin, and statins. What came out on top? Smoking cessation! Aspirin was the second most cost-effective treatment, and blood pressure medicines were third. Statins were dead last.[25]

So what should you do? Should you take them? Ditch them?

The answer: It's complicated.

If you already have heart disease, statins are probably a good idea, especially if you tolerate them and experience no undesirable side effects. I do suggest statins to my heart patients, in lower doses, sometimes only three to four times a week, and always with the CoQ10 supplemental program. Talk to your health care provider about such an approach. It might very well allow you to have the benefit of statin therapy without the downside of muscle weakness, pain, and other health problems. For more on CoQ10, see page 256 in Chapter 11.

Also, make sure to pair statin therapy with a heart-healthy lifestyle, the very same lifestyle I promote on every page of this book.

Statins can certainly help heart patients with very high cholesterol LDL particle numbers, but the only way to truly protect your heart—and also be able to avoid medication-induced side effects—is to incorporate as many lifestyle prescriptions into your daily repertoire as possible while you take your necessary prescription medications.

Beta-Blockers

Another common class of prescription medications for heart patients is beta-blockers, which lower blood pressure by blocking the effects of the hormone epinephrine (also called adrenaline). When you take them, your heart beats more slowly and with less force. Older brands still used include metoprolol (Lopressor or Toprol), acebutolol (Sectral), atenolol (Tenormin), bisoprolol (Zebeta), nadolol (Corgard), and several others.

Although these medicines have been shown to reduce the risk of death after a heart attack for one to seven years, they are not the answer for most patients. Here's why: Many beta-blockers can elevate blood sugar and alter cholesterol numbers unfavorably. That's rather disappointing. In the past, it was common to place patients on a beta-blocker in the hope that it would prevent a first attack, but newer data has called this practice into question. Unless you have chest pain (angina), high blood pressure, or heart rhythm abnormalities, taking a beta-blocker probably offers you little help and may actually be a detriment if yours is one of the brands that adversely affects blood sugar and cholesterol numbers. Older beta-blockers also commonly cause fatigue, cold extremities, and depression.

When I treat patients who have suffered a heart attack, I almost exclusively use carvedilol, a generic beta-blocker that has favorable effects on blood sugar and cholesterol profiles. In addition, carvedilol has strong antioxidant properties and acts like a combination beta-blocker and multivitamin. It has been shown to have favorable effects after heart attacks, in congestive heart failure, and for high blood pressure. If you've already suffered a heart attack and are on a beta-blocker, talk to your health care provider about possibly switching to this particular brand. If you are taking a beta-blocker, please do not stop without discussing this with your health care provider.

ACE Inhibitors

Another medication that has impressive data in heart patients and heart attack survivors is the group of drugs called ACE inhibitors. ACE stands for "angiotensin-converting enzyme," and these medications block that enzyme from narrowing your blood vessels and releasing hormones that spike blood pressure.

There are many different brands of ACE inhibitors including benazepril (Lotensin), enalapril (Vasotec), lisinopil (Prinivil), and several others. When used, these medications can drop blood pressure, reduce the severity of congestive heart failure, and allow the heart to heal more completely after a heart attack. They may actually slow down the aging of arteries, too.

After decades of use the only common side effect from these drugs is a dry cough.

Although the main use of ACE inhibitors has been for people with elevated blood pressure, a landmark study called the HOPE trial examined the impact of prescribing an ACE inhibitor to heart disease patients with normal blood pressure. When researchers found that overall death rates, heart deaths, heart attacks, and the need for angioplasty or bypass surgery were all significantly lower in patients taking ramipril (Altace), compared to those on a placebo, they halted the study early so they could allow those on the placebo to have access to this lifesaving medicine.

As an added benefit, patients taking ACE inhibitors have a lower risk of developing diabetes and a slower progression of calcified plaque in coronary arteries.

Because of the HOPE trial, I do select ramipril for my patients over other ACE inhibitors. Ramipril has the advantage of blocking ACE in both kidneys and the actual walls of arteries (a tissue ACE inhibitor), and may slow the hardening of arteries found with age. Many experts consider ACE inhibitors a routine part of an anti-aging program in anyone with any signs of vascular disease. I agree with this. If a dry cough develops on ACE inhibitors, a similar group of compounds called ARBs (angiotensin receptor blockers) is available.

I just made ACE inhibitors sound like an amazing invention and truly they are. So why are *they* not the answer? As with any drug, if you take them without changing your lifestyle, you are treating only one small part of a body-wide problem. *To truly halt heart disease and extend your life, you must pair a heart-healthy lifestyle with the best of prescription meds.* Or, as I like to say, always take this medication with food and exercise—vegetables, fruits, and walking, for example. I even recommend walking to the drugstore.

WHY ANGIOPLASTY AND STENTING AREN'T THE ANSWER

In the 1970s, there was a revolution in the treatment of heart disease. European physician Andreas Gruentzig, MD, stood in his kitchen and began a side project. He thought that if he could build a balloon that was both sturdy and incredibly small, he could attach it to a catheter and thread it into a blood vessel in someone's leg and then up their body until he got to the main arteries that led to the heart. There he would inject fluid into the catheter and inflate the balloon. If he did this over and over again, the balloon would flatten plaque (much like stomping on fresh snow) and

---

Ask the Holistic Heart Doc:

I can't tolerate statins. Is there anything else I can try?

Yes, there is! I've had many heart disease patients who can't tolerate routine doses of statins because of muscle aching or memory loss. For these patients I prescribe a plant-based diet coupled with one or more of the following supplements that work to drive down cholesterol and reduce inflammation, but without the unfortunate side effects:

Plant sterols: 2 grams a day.

Tocotrienols (a type of vitamin E): 200 mg at night.

Pantethine (a form of vitamin B_5): 450 mg twice a day.

Green tea extracts (EGCG): 500 mg twice a day.

High-quality forms of red yeast rice: up to 4,800 mg at night.

Niacin (vitamin B_3): up to 2 to 3 grams a day.

Omega-3 fatty acids: up to 4 grams a day.

Berberine: 500 mg twice a day.

I've also found that many of the unfortunate side effects of statins can be eliminated just by reducing the dose. Most patients experience no side effects when they take statins just one to three times a week at lower doses. For example, rosuvastatin (Crestor) 10 mg just twice a week might drop the LDL cholesterol by 15 to 20 percent without the side effects. Also, switching brands might help. Pitavastatin (Livalo) lowers levels of CoQ10 less than other statins. I have used this medication with much success, even in many patients who were considered untreatable with other statin brands. I always combine statins with CoQ10 supplements, usually 200 to 400 mg daily.

---

compact it into a hard pancake. The end result? Arteries could be widened and cleared of obstructions without surgery.

Once he developed a prototype, he tested it in animals and then in humans. When he passed the balloon catheter into a blocked area and inflated the balloon, it did exactly as he had suspected. It reduced the amount of narrowing in the vessel. The now wider artery provided more blood flow, and angina (chest pain) symptoms, shortness of breath, and abnormal stress tests were resolved.

He called this invention percutaneous transluminal coronary angioplasty (PTCA), or angioplasty for short. A few years later my mentor, Geoffrey Hartzler, MD, in Kansas City, began using PTCA in patients with multiple blockages, and even in patients who were having a heart attack, pushing the field far ahead and competing head on with bypass surgery, developed a decade earlier.

The industry and the number of PTCA procedures grew phenomenally during the 1980s and early 1990s but the limitations in angioplasty were obvious. Within just six to nine months, nearly half of all arteries treated with PTCA closed back up. Also, five percent of the time PTCA would injure the artery and emergency and very risky bypass surgery was needed.

In the early 1990s a strategy to deal with complications and re-narrowing of the blood vessels was developed by a radiologist in Texas, Julio Palmaz, MD. He showed that, after using the balloon to widen the artery, stainless steel coils called stents could be inserted to prop the artery open. The stents reduced the need for emergency surgery and also cut the rate of restenosis down significantly. (Dr. Palmaz created the first stent models from chicken wire he noticed behind his drywall during a kitchen renovation!)

But there still remained drawbacks. The first models were stiff and hard to insert, and plaque and tissue often still grew back, closing the artery back up. Over the years, however, better designs helped improve the long-term success rate. Stents became more flexible and thinner, and were coated with drugs that prevented tissue re-growth. These drugs were much like weed killers;

they kept the cells from reacting to the metal and growing through the openings in the mesh stents to re-narrow the artery.

So, you're wondering, if they've improved so much, why aren't they the answer? Let us count the ways:

A year is a long time to be on a blood thinner. After you've had a stent inserted, you'll need to take two blood-thinning pills (aspirin and another drug such as clopidogrel or prasugrel) for at least a year. This is called DAPT or dual anti-platelet therapy. I call this blood thinner prison because patients with drug-coated stents cannot undergo any procedure that might induce bleeding during the entire time they are on these blood thinners. If they must undergo a procedure—such as a biopsy or repair of a broken bone—they either have to discontinue the blood thinners first, at high risk of the stents clotting, or delay the procedure, hampering diagnosis and treatment.

They don't extend your life. Studies of routinely scheduled stent procedures generally show no advantage in life span when compared to cardiac exercise programs and lifestyle changes.

Stents only treat one small area of your body. Stents are usually less than an inch long, and at most 1.5 inches. On the other hand, the arteries that feed the heart are nearly 20 inches long. Your stent might do a great job of keeping one inch of that 20-inch-long tube open, but the rest of the tube might already have mild plaque and be 25 to 50 percent clogged—even on the day of your procedure. If you do nothing to stop the onward march of clogged arteries, you may need another and another and another stent, until you have a "full metal jacket" coating your arteries. If you were ever to need a bypass surgery, this could hamper the surgeon's success.

Now, stents do save lives, especially if they are inserted into patients who are having active heart attacks. When such a patient comes to the emergency room, a whole team of medical personnel works to transfer him or her to the cardiac catheterization laboratory as soon as possible. In these patients, an artery can be completely blocked, and PTCA and stenting truly save lives.

Another good reason to stent is if you have very abnormal stress

Ask the Holistic Heart Doc:

Are there any office procedures that can help me avoid a bypass or angioplasty?

Yes, and I highly recommend you ask your cardiologist about it before undergoing the knife or balloon. A treatment called external counter pulsation (ECP) could very well keep you out of the surgical suite.

A number of years ago Chinese investigators discovered a way to provide intermittent pressure to the body externally—without the need for surgery. The technique, ECP, helps boost blood flow and heart performance. I am proud to have brought the first ECP machine to Michigan years ago.

To undergo the treatment, you just lie on a padded table one hour a day, five days a week, for seven weeks, for a total of 35 hours of therapy. During this hour the console provides intermittent inflation and deflation to pressure cuffs placed around the legs and hips. When researchers compared the ECP treatment to a sham procedure where the cuffs where not really inflated, ECP resulted in fewer episodes of angina, fewer requirements for nitroglycerin tablets sublingually for the treatment of angina, improved stamina, and actually smaller areas of poor blood flow on heart scans. The treatment really works! After 35 hours of therapy, the improvement is often sustained for months, or even years. Scientists think that new blood vessels called collaterals may form from ECP therapy and improvement in endothelial function results.

Ask your cardiologist about this treatment, especially if:

- You have chest pain that isn't responding to lifestyle changes or medications.

- Angioplasty or stenting is being recommended to a small branch vessel.

- You have a totally blocked heart artery.

The widely available therapy can be repeated at any time, and often just a few weeks of repeated ECP treatment can yield sustained results. Insurance programs usually will pay for this proven therapy.

tests showing large areas of poor blood flow that put your heart at risk. Similarly, if you have angina pectoris (chest pain) that hasn't responded to medication, angioplasty and stenting might be the answer. This is particularly true if the angina discomfort is coming on more frequently or lasting longer.

Stents are amazing for unstable patients at risk of or having a heart attack, but for the rest of us the answer is: Meditate, don't medicate! And if you've already had a stent? It's just as important to practice heart-healthy lifestyle changes so you can prevent the need for another stent. As I say, "Prevent, don't stent."

WHY YOU WANT TO BYPASS BYPASS SURGERY

Coronary artery bypass graft (CABG) surgery was developed in the late 1960s by an innovative surgeon at the Cleveland Clinic. By the time angioplasty was introduced, bypass surgery was the established remedy for blocked arteries that did not respond to medication. It took decades to determine that, for most patients, angioplasty and stents had the same long-term safety and survival results as bypass surgery—and with less pain, suffering, and recovery time.

If most people knew exactly what bypass surgery entailed along with the data on the long-term success rates, it's my belief that the vast majority of them would do everything possible to prevent ever having to undergo such an operation by changing their lifestyle. So, please bear with me while I explain this operation in excruciating detail. That way you'll have more motivation than ever to incorporate as many heart-friendly changes as possible into your life as early as possible.

This, folks, is quite possibly the most extensive operation a human could ever undergo. A typical bypass surgery lasts two to four hours. A surgeon will saw the chest bone in two and use a bone spreader on the ribs, much as a firefighter uses the jaws of life to wedge open a car.

While some bypass surgeries are now done on beating hearts, most are not. Once the chest is opened large tubes nearly the size of garden hoses are inserted into the red blood aorta and the blue blood veins to divert the blood to a machine that will pump oxygenated blood throughout the body. Then, in many cases, surgeons will stop the heart with a potassium-based mixture and cover it in ice, hoping to preserve it while working on it in a pause mode.

As this is going on, a second team of surgeons or assistants works down at the end of the table to "harvest" a length of vein from a leg. Veins were not meant to carry red blood, but there are simply not enough arteries in your body for surgeons to use them for the typical triple or quadruple bypass, so leg veins usually get dragged into the procedure. Some surgeons do try to use only artery bypasses by borrowing them from the wrist or the stomach, but this is uncommon. Usually, the surgeons make small incisions up and down the leg, snaking out a section of vein and placing it in a bowl.

Then surgeons sew pieces of the vein to arteries near the heart to redirect blood around blockages. The more blockages, the more veins are sewed in. Once all is done, the heart is shocked back to life, the ribs are pressed back together, the chest bone is wired and glued, and the patient is put into the intensive care unit.

Patients who undergo a bypass will miss work for usually a minimum of about two months. That's an incredibly long recovery. The sternal bone doesn't heal for six weeks, so driving and lifting are prohibited for that amount of time. Sometimes the bone does not heal completely. Called a non-union, this results in a clicking sound and unstable motion of the chest results.

Depending on the size, number, and location of blockages, it's possible that a newer, minimally invasive bypass surgery approach may be used. Minimally invasive surgery does not involve sawing open the chest. Instead, surgeons access the arteries through smaller incisions or with the assistance of robotic systems but may not be able to reach all targets if there are multiple blockages.

I always wonder what would have happened if angioplasty had been developed before bypass surgery. If it was already the established practice to treat heart disease through a small poke through the skin in the groin or arm, would anyone have taken to the idea of putting a person to sleep, cracking open the chest, stopping the heart, cutting the legs, sewing the veins around the arteries, putting in chest tubes, and requiring patients to stay in the ICU and the hospital for up to a week? I doubt it, except in rare instances.

Now, all of that said, bypass surgery can be lifesaving. Who might need one? Some patients have such extensive heart disease that no amount of medication, external counter pulsation, and/or stenting could overcome it. If your cardiologist tells you that you have severe disease in all three heart artcrics (or even just in the left main artery) that is unreachable with a stent, a bypass just might be your best and possibly only option. These are among the only patterns of heart disease that have shown a long-term benefit of bypass surgery over medications, external counter pulsation, or stents.

I hope, however, that you now agree with me that a bypass is not something you want to undergo if you can help it. And if you've already had a bypass, you are not cured of your heart disease. *In fact, if you've had a bypass, it's even more important to practice the prescriptions in this book.* Here's why:

Veins don't last forever. The vein bypasses from the leg have a finite life span. These blood vessels just are not designed to be cut out, moved, and used to carry arterial high-pressure blood. As many as 10 to 20 percent of these vein bypass grafts become completely closed just one year after surgery, in some cases, resulting in chest pain, heart damage, additional procedures, or medications. Some close up just a month after the operation! Think about that. It takes at least two months to completely recover. Before you've even returned to work, some of those veins might already be totally and permanently clogged. That's not a very good return for your pain and suffering investment. It is not uncommon for someone to have a quadruple bypass (usually three vein pieces and one artery piece used for the bridges) and find out within a few years of the operation that all the veins are shut and only one artery bypass is still open.

Bypass does not solve the underlying problem. Does bypass surgery lower your cholesterol, blood sugar, blood pressure, or inflammation? Does it remove toxins from your body? Does it counteract the effects of smoking, air pollution, and a bad diet? Does it stop the stress that raises levels of hormones that are just as destructive to your arteries as high cholesterol? Does it improve sleep and give your body a chance to repair itself?

In a word: no.

Like stents, bypass surgery is a bandage for a problem that needs long-term, body-wide treatment. It does nothing to prevent the development of new blockages.

Once you've had one bypass, you'll never ask for another. Must I say more? A bypass is the kind of operation that most people are simply glad to have survived and lived to tell about. No one wants another one, but some need it if not attending to their healthy habits.

If you are recovering from stenting or bypass surgery, be grateful for the technology that provided new blood flow to your heart muscles, but don't buy into that false sense of security. You are not cured. You've only been given a second chance to wake up and grasp on to true heart health via changes in your diet, your movement, and other lifestyle measures. Rather than relax and maintain the same lifestyle that clogged your arteries in the first place, emulate former president Bill Clinton.

A few years after his bypass surgery, he was floored when he learned that he had lost a bypass graft and required a stent. Searching for real answers to preventing more problems, he sought out Dr. Caldwell Esselstyn of the Cleveland Clinic. Once he was schooled in the research and strategy for eating a very low-fat, plant-based diet, Clinton lost weight, gained vitality, and is looking years younger. He learned how to say no to things harming his heart and a big yes to things healing his arteries.

You can do the same, by using the prescriptions in this book!

WHY A HEART-HEALTHY LIFESTYLE IS THE TRUE ANSWER

No matter where you are on the heart disease continuum—whether you simply want to prevent a strong family history from sealing your fate or even whether you've already suffered a heart attack—a heart-healthy lifestyle is your true answer.

If you wish to live a long, healthy, and happy life, you'll want to incorporate every single option available to protect and heal arteries

---

Ask the Holistic Heart Doc:
My arteries are only 50 percent blocked. What does that mean?

It means that you want to do everything you can to keep your arteries from getting fully blocked, and you need to do it right now in hopes that you can reverse the disease process.

Do you think an artery that became 100 percent blocked and led to a heart attack was 90 percent blocked a few months before? Or do you think it was perhaps 30 to 50 percent blocked before and got worse rapidly, even in minutes? When a Danish cardiologist by the name of Ehrling Falk, MD, examined this question he found, to the surprise of most people in the medical field, that 68 percent of the time the totally blocked artery was less than 50 percent blocked on the earlier angiogram and only 32 percent of the time was it more than 50 percent blocked.

Rapid progression of blockages, like a volcano beginning to erupt, is felt to be common before a big heart attack. This is important because in the past many people with arteries that were 25 to 50 percent blocked were told that they had nothing to worry about. That is usually heard by the patient as, "I do not need to make changes in my lifestyle." In fact, these early blockages greatly respond to lifestyle changes. Do not be lax about the changes you need to make. You can guard yourself against heart attacks and strokes.

and preserve heart function. Low-fat, plant-based diets have been proven to reverse heart disease. Lowering your intake of animal fat and protein, reducing your exposure to toxins, and consuming the highest concentration of vegetable super healers (phytonutrients that fight for your health), plant fiber, and minerals gives you the greatest chance of arresting and reversing arterial blockages.

Do you think this sounds too hard? I hope, by now, I've convinced you that bypass surgery is what's hard. Hospital admissions are hard. Strokes are hard. Erectile dysfunction (a common side effect of heart disease) is hard (sort of). Taking 11 medications every day is hard. Injecting insulin into your abdomen is hard. Death is hard.

Learning to eat and move in a heart-healthy way? When you compare it to your alternative, it comes out sounding downright easy.

I'd like to end this chapter by telling you a story. In the 1950s, Nathan Pritikin read about a doctor in California who was successfully treating his heart disease patients with a diet that resembled World War II rations. The portions were meager. Fat and cholesterol were low. Plants were eaten at every meal and made up most of the diet. And the cholesterol levels of his patients had all dropped an average of 100 points.

Pritikin's own blood cholesterol topped 300 mg/dl, but he was attached to his three-egg breakfast, his nightly pint of ice cream, and his generous usage of butter and whipped cream. Then, at age 41, he learned that his arteries were clogged. He was having angina chest pressure as a warning of an impending heart attack. Although he was an engineer (and not a doctor), he studied the science of heart disease and decided to make some major changes in his lifestyle.

He stopped eating meat of all kinds, he added in a rainbow of plant-based foods, and he started running three to four miles a day. Within months he'd slashed his cholesterol level in half. He stopped having chest pain. His abnormal stress test became normal. He later wrote a bestselling book describing his regimen and established the Pritikin Longevity Center to share this breakthrough with others. Years later when he died due to complications of leukemia, an autopsy demonstrated that he now had exceptionally clean heart arteries a full 30 years after he'd been diagnosed with clogged ones.

His story shows that you can not only stop heart disease, you can reverse it, and you can do it just with some diet and lifestyle changes, some of the very changes you'll find showcased in this book. You can be just like Nathan Pritikin. The whole heart prescriptions in Part Two will—one small change at a time—help you to adopt a heart-healing diet similar to the one Pritikin followed and advocated. In addition, you'll gain important recommendations for fitness, stress relief, and clean, toxin-free living that Pritikin didn't know about, but probably would be promoting were he still alive today.

It doesn't matter how high your blood cholesterol, blood pressure, or blood sugar are right now. It doesn't matter how many medications you are on or how many symptoms you have.

You can turn this around, and you can make the biggest impact not with drugs and not with surgery, but rather with everyday tools you'll find in your own home, tools as simple as a fork and a pair of walking shoes.

Heart disease is curable. It can be reversed, and it can be prevented, too.

It is within your control.

You are not helpless. You have so many tools at your disposal. The body is capable of healing itself. Remove the ingredients for disease and replace them with ingredients for health, and I guarantee you will see your vitality return and, like Nathan Pritikin and so many others, you will defy the odds.

Chapter 4

Score Your Heart

How old is your heart? If you are like many people, then the first number that comes to mind is probably the number of years you've been on the planet. So, if you are 40 years old, you assume your heart is 40 years old, too.

In reality, your heart might be older or younger than the number of years you've lived. If you come from a family with strong, healthy hearts and you've treated your heart with care, your ticker might behave as if it's five, 10, 15, or even 20 years younger than the number of candles on your birthday cake. On the other hand, if you come from a family riddled with heart disease and you've fed your heart a steady diet of stress, toxins, and junk food, your heart might be much older than your physical age.

Indeed, your heart's true age depends both on your genetics (what you inherited from your parents) and your lifestyle (what you did with what you inherited), as well as your environmental exposure. You can't go back and choose different parents, but you can definitely do something about your lifestyle and environmental exposure. And the amazing news is this: By changing your lifestyle, you really can grow younger, healthier, and happier. What you do matters a lot—a lot more than most people think.

THE NUDGE WE ALL NEED

We all have the power to add years to our lives, yet many of us squander it. Rather than consume heart-healthy foods, we find ourselves continually attracted to cheese puffs, fried dough, and soft drinks. Rather than do something about our tension, we keep telling ourselves, "I'll get on that tomorrow." But we never do. It's the same with exercise.

Why? Chances are, it's a false sense of security. You can't see heart disease. For many years, you can't feel it, either. Yet, much like a stealthy ninja, it's been there, hiding in the darkness, and silently getting worse for years.

This is true even if you have zero symptoms and feel great. It's true even if your health care provider has placed a stethoscope to your chest and could not hear anything out of the ordinary. It's even true if you've had normal test results for an electrocardiogram (ECG), a standard cholesterol panel, or an exercise stress test.

Since you've undergone testing and your health care provider has given you the "all clear," you subconsciously think "it's not a big deal, I'm okay," whenever you eat a bag of fried snack chips or grab a doughnut and a whipped-cream-and-sugar-loaded coffee drink and rush to work. It's the same with spending all evening in front of the TV.

But it is a big deal and you probably aren't okay. If you didn't already at least partially believe this, you wouldn't be reading this book. Still, you're probably wondering: How could my health care provider be wrong? How could so many tests be wrong?

As I mentioned in Chapter 2, heart disease is complex. The entire body affects the heart and, everyday, we're learning that one aspect of heart health—such as your total cholesterol levels—can appear exceptionally healthy while another aspect of heart health (such as the functioning of the endothelial lining of your arteries) can be anything but.

If you knew without a doubt that you not only had heart disease, but that the problem was slowly and surely getting worse, you'd probably feel very motivated to do something about it, wouldn't you? Rather than thinking, "I need to do something about my lifestyle at some point," you'd tell yourself, "I need to change my lifestyle today—right now!" Well, let's all wake up and vote YES for healthy hearts.

It's my hope that this chapter will bring you to that "right now!" place. In the following pages you'll learn about several self-assessments and office tests. The office tests are the cutting edge. Not all physicians offer them, and insurance doesn't cover some of them. Yet they are the best way to shock yourself out of this false sense of health and, finally, detect this silent killer so you can motivate yourself to do something about it.

ASSESS YOUR HEALTH AT HOME

The quick-scoring examination I suggest in this section is not anywhere near as accurate or enlightening as true diagnostic tests your health care provider can do in the office or hospital with the most modern heart disease detectors. Still, it can, at the very least, give you the incentive to make an appointment. Use your answers to the following questions to get an idea of the silent disease you might want to know more about.

Evaluate your risk factors. Many different diseases, lifestyle habits, and inherited conditions dramatically raise your risk of developing heart disease. Look at the following list. Give yourself 2 points for every statement that is true for you:

* You've already been diagnosed with diabetes, high blood pressure, or very high cholesterol (>250 mg/dl) or obesity.

* You are a postmenopausal woman or had a hysterectomy at a young age.

* You are a man over 40 or a woman over 55.

* You smoke or quit smoking in the last five years.

* You work a desk job.

* You don't exercise.

* You drink one or more soft drinks a day.

* You feel tension and stress on a regular basis.

* You sleep fewer than 6 hours at night.

* You have a family history of heart disease.

* You have few friends, social connections, or support groups.

If you scored 4 or higher, then don't think of the prescriptions in this book as "something I'll get to when I have more time." Consider them doctor's orders. The subtlest lifestyle habits, repeated day after day, month after month, year after year can eventually land you in the hospital with a case of sudden-onset chest pain. Don't let that happen to you. Even if you feel great now, your lifestyle could be eroding your health.

If you scored 6 or higher, I highly encourage you to visit your health care provider and ask about the office tests outlined in the next section.

Check your symptoms. It can take many years for heart disease to bring on obvious symptoms like chest pain. If you know how to interpret them, however, you can spot the signs of impending heart disease quite early. One of the first signs of heart disease affects your sex life. I mentioned the importance of the hormone testosterone for men in Chapter 2. Men with lower testosterone levels tend to develop heart disease and die at a younger age than men with normal levels. And low testosterone tends to show up as erectile dysfunction. Similarly, the blood vessels that lead to the penis tend to clog earlier than the ones that lead to the heart. Whether due to vascular issues or testosterone deficiency, erectile dysfunction can serve as an important clue that heart disease is silently developing. Get checked!

Another sign of heart disease, especially in women: fatigue, especially if it comes on with exertion. Even if the fatigue seems benign—for instance, you feel especially tired at the end of a light exercise session or after doing some housework—get checked. It might be your heart or it might be issues with another organ, such as your thyroid. Either way, don't ignore it and don't minimize it. Tell your health care provider. Even significant balding on the top of the head or a diagonal deep crease on your earlobe can be a sign of early heart disease that ought not be ignored.

And, I hope it goes without saying: If you experience *any* shortness of breath or chest pressure, seek medical attention. This is a sign that your heart disease has come out of hiding. Don't ignore it! Chest pressure or shortness of breath on exertion, such as carrying a heavy garbage can out to the curb in cold weather or dragging a laundry basket up the stairs from the basement, generally means that the heart is starving. This is called angina pectoris (chest pain), and usually does not happen until your arteries are more than 70 percent blocked. If you are having any of these problems, please see your health care provider right away.

TESTS TO ASK YOUR DOCTOR ABOUT

It's my hope that the previous section provided you with a strong incentive to see your health care provider. When you do visit your physician, don't settle for the usual once-over. As I mentioned, it's easy for health care providers to miss heart disease, especially if their diagnostic tests involve a stethoscope, an ECG, and a cholesterol panel. This is especially true in women. Unfortunately, for many women, a heart attack is their first indication that something is wrong.

So take this book with you to the doctor's office and ask about the following tests. Not all of them are covered by insurance, but that doesn't make them any less important than the typical tests your health care provider performs. They are all well worth the out-of-pocket expense.

I call these SHARK detectors because they spot Silent Heart Attack Risk Killers. Just as, during an otherwise relaxing ocean swim, a shark can come up without warning and surprise you with a serious attack, so can a silent heart blockage. These tests help you to see the SHARK long before it surfaces, giving you plenty of time to get yourself out of dangerous waters.

SHARK Detector #1: Coronary Artery Calcium Scoring (CACS)

When most people think of calcium, they think of bones. That's probably because 99 percent of the body's calcium is stored in bone. But calcium is also found in other places, including the blood vessels. Tiny amounts of calcium are floating through your blood at this very moment. And while calcium is good for your bones, it's not so good for the lining of your blood vessels.

Just as calcium hardens your bones, it can also harden your blood vessels, causing your blood vessels to stiffen. Stiff blood vessels make it harder for your heart to pump blood where it needs to go. This drives pressure up, which, in turn, makes it more likely that particles in the blood (especially the golf-ball-like small, dense LDL cholesterol) stick to the lining of the arteries, damaging them and setting the stage for dangerous plaque to form.

You need calcium in your blood to help charge the many reactions inside of your cells, but you don't want calcium deposits in the linings of your arteries. Calcium scoring using a CT or CAT scan to detect the hardness of your heart arteries helps detect levels of calcium in the lining of the blood vessels. The science in support of CT heart calcium scoring has skyrocketed. *More than 1,000 studies show that calcium scoring is one of the most powerful screening tools for silent heart disease.* It's truly the best SHARK test around. So why haven't you heard about it? Why haven't you had one? Beats me! I talk about it all the time on TV and radio and recommend it to patients all the time. I have ordered and interpreted thousands of these scans for patients.

How the test works. A CT scan detects the calcium in your heart blood vessels. These special "multi-slice" machines are available at most hospitals and some physician offices. All you have to do is find a machine, lie down for a moment or two, and hold your breath.

What your score means. The ideal score is zero. If your score is between 1 and 10, be very motivated to change your lifestyle. If you score between 11 and 100, get serious about learning more about heart disease prevention and making some changes. If you score between 100 and 400+, follow up with a stress test, take a serious look at your habits, and make a commitment to change many of them to prevent and reverse this coating of bone in your heart pipes.

Who should have it done. The American College of Cardiology strongly recommends this exam for anyone with some risk for early heart disease. Because this test delivers a dose of radiation, however, hold off until you are 50 or older, unless you have a major risk factor for heart disease such as a strong family history of early heart disease, are a smoker, or have diabetes. I ask all my healthy patients by age 50 to consider scheduling this exam to check their heart arteries.

How often to have it done. I do not repeat calcium scoring if it is abnormal. Once you know you have heart disease, use that as motivation. Tape the test result to your refrigerator and your gym shoes. You don't need to keep doing the test to see how much worse your calcium score is getting. If your calcium score is zero, wait a decade before repeating the test to avoid excessive radiation. I did my own checkup at age 50 and had a score of zero. I don't plan to undergo the test again until I turn 60.

The cost. Most insurance companies do not cover this screening exam, but many hospitals now charge only $100 or less for it. Call around. Some hospitals charge much more than others. On the other hand, I know of a local hospital where the test is only $48.

Limitations. Any CT scan will deliver a dose of radiation, which can raise your risk of other diseases, especially cancer. Newer scanners are faster, have special protective software programs, and expose you to much lower doses of radiation. Still, I don't recommend the test for people under age 45, unless they are heavy smokers, have long-term diabetes, have very high cholesterol of 300 mg/dl or more or have a strong family history of early heart disease. Never undergo calcium scoring (or any other test that delivers radiation) if you are pregnant.

You might be able to lessen the damage from calcium scoring and other X-rays by loading up on foods rich in antioxidant vitamins in the days before.

The other limitation is that some artery plaques don't calcify. That means, even if you have a calcium score of zero, you might still have some plaque. There are very few plaques like this, however, and these softer types of plaques generally do not progress to heart attacks. If you have chest pain or any other symptom that leads you to suspect you have blocked arteries, don't allow a calcium score of zero to give you a false sense of security. Definitely follow up with other tests.

SHARK Detector #2: Carotid Intimal Medial Thickness (CIMT)

There is another simple technique for finding silent artery disease. This one uses an ultrasound machine to see inside the major carotid artery in the neck. This artery connects the heart to the brain. When it's diseased, it's very likely that other arteries inside your body are also diseased.

How the test works. The ultrasound shows the thickness of the inner two linings of the wall of the artery (called the intima and media). If these walls are getting too thick, it's a sign of early atherosclerosis. The advantage of CIMT is that it uses ultrasound so there is no radiation risk. The exam is painless and usually takes under 15 minutes with results immediately available.

What your results mean. If the CIMT is in a normal range (approximately 0.7 mm or less based on age or a thin artery wall), the risk of blockages anywhere in the body—including the heart—is very low. If the CIMT is abnormal (0.8 mm and up), the silent killer is working slowly to harm you and it is time to make over your lifestyle! The thicker the lining of your carotid arteries, the more plaque and the higher the risk of future heart attack and stroke.

Who should have it done. This test has received a high recommendation from the American College of Cardiology, and there are more than 500 scientific studies that speak to its effectiveness. I recommend it to most patients once they reach the age of 50, but often even earlier for people who smoke, have high cholesterol, or a family history of vascular disease. Because no radiation is involved, there is no health risk, so the test can be used in younger patients with confidence. Surprisingly, it's still not widely available.

How often to repeat the test. If you can afford it, repeat the test as often as every six months to a year to see if your prevention program is working.

The cost. CIMT is only covered by some insurance plans and only in a few locations. Clinics charge between $150 and $250 on average, but the test is well worth the expense.

Limitations. While many physicians and health care centers own the equipment to do a CIMT, they don't all have the special software package that is needed to measure the thickness of the carotid artery and compare it to a normal thickness. To make sure your test is useful, ask if your hospital, clinic, or health care provider will be doing the test using special software dedicated for measuring CIMT. Unfortunately, the cost of the test can be out of range for some people, especially if their insurance doesn't cover it.

SHARK Detector #3: EndoPAT

You already learned that arteries are lined with a single layer of super cells called the endothelium. These cells keep the artery resistant to injury and clotting, and also allow the arteries to relax (or dilate) to provide more blood flow when needed.

Healthy arteries spring back quickly after being squeezed, for instance, by a blood pressure cuff. Once the cuff is removed, blood flow doubles, triples, or even quadruples for a few seconds to minutes. Diseased arteries don't do this. Blood flow only very slowly comes back. When blood vessels don't spring back, it is a sign called endothelial dysfunction.

Endothelial dysfunction is one of the earliest signs of artery disease that we are capable of detecting.

How the test works. The EndoPAT is a device made in Israel, and more than 200 studies support its use. It no longer considered experimental, and is now approved for use in many countries. A blood pressure cuff is placed on an arm and is inflated for five minutes, while a special clip is placed on one finger of each hand. When the cuff suddenly releases, the blood flow should increase greatly in the hand that was starving for blood (the one with the cuffed arm), but not on the hand that was not. When researchers from the Mayo Clinic did this test on more than 250 people and then tracked their health outcomes for six years, the study participants with a poor blood flow had a higher risk of heart attack or death. The researchers concluded that EndoPAT testing could predict which patients were likely to suffer chest pain, heart attack, and other undesirable outcomes.[26]

What your score means. Your EndoScore is usually calculated immediately during the visit. Anything more than 2 means your arteries are responding in a healthy manner and your endothelial lining is working. If the number is below 1.67, there is definitely a problem and intensive changes in lifestyle (again, eating better, stress management, supplements, and the many other suggestions in this book) are needed.

Who should have it done. I recommend EndoPAT for people who just want to know where they stand, but also for those who already know they have heart disease. Even if you've already had a stent inserted or bypass surgery, this test can help motivate you to get your lifestyle back to being as heart healthy as possible. With hard work, you can heal the inner lining of your arteries, making them much less likely to reclog. A patient with a stent who has a normal EndoScore is much healthier than a similar patient with a poor EndoScore.

How often to repeat the test. I have patients repeat the exam every six months, or until their endothelial function returns to normal. Then I have them repeat it once a year. It can take months for lifestyle changes to reverse endothelial dysfunction, but they really do work. I've seen it happen for my patients. It is a great feeling to know that the artery lining has healed.

Costs. The test costs under $200, but it's covered by most insurance plans.

Limitations. It's possible to have full-blown heart artery disease (and even to have undergone bypass surgery or stenting) and have normal endothelial function. This means that your arteries have some plaque, but the lining is healthy. This is a good place to be for a heart patient, but it doesn't mean you should ignore lifestyle changes.

SHARK Detector #4: Advanced Blood Tests

At a yearly visit with your family practitioner or internist, you will likely get a fasting blood sugar and cholesterol profile. These tests are great, but, as I've mentioned, they miss a lot. Many people who have suffered from heart attacks did so after passing a "standard examination" in the years before and with completely normal levels of total cholesterol. The good news: The same vials of blood can tell you and your health care provider so much more about your health, assuming your health care provider asks the lab for the information. If you're going to let someone draw blood and examine it, you might as well learn as much as you can in the process. So during your annual screening, talk to your health care provider about having the lab check your blood for at least some of the following:

Advanced cholesterol panel. You've probably been told to keep your total cholesterol below 200 and your LDL cholesterol below 130 mg/dl. In addition to knowing that information, you also want to know the LDL particle number and size (remember the minivans versus small cars I mentioned in the previous chapter).

High-sensitivity C-reactive protein. In Chapter 2, I told you about inflammation, the fire that slowly erodes blood vessels and other organs in the body. C-reactive protein is a marker for inflammation. In the past decade, a test for high-sensitivity C-reactive protein (hs-CRP) has changed the assessment of patients dramatically. If your hs-CRP is normal (usually <1.0 mg/dl), your arteries do not appear to be inflamed by your diet, lifestyle, or other factors. On the other hand, if your hs-CRP is elevated (anything from 1 mg/dl all the way to over 20), something is wrong with your lifestyle or health and major efforts to identify and correct problems need to be pursued. I order this exam on every patient at least once a year. If the results are abnormal, I go over diet and exercise solutions as well as search for unexpected sites of inflammation including dental, prostate, urinary, and bowel infections that may uncover a subtle root cause.

Homocysteine. About 40 years ago an astute doctor observed early artery damage in young children who had an elevated level of a naturally occurring amino acid called homocysteine. Research led to identifying a very complex series of chemical reactions in the body that deal with amino acid metabolism (a process called methylation) and certain vitamins that make these cycles hum. In adults, increased levels of homocysteine have also been associated with increased risk of vascular damage. At a minimum this test reflects the status of the methylation process in the body, so it's a very important way to regulate gene function. Patients with high levels of homocysteine can be treated with B complex vitamins, which is a pretty simple solution. A safe homocysteine level is under 10 µmol/l (micromoles per liter) and even better levels read under 8 µmol/l. I get very concerned when it is in the high teens or over 20 µmol/l. When the homocysteine is very high,

Ask the Holistic Heart Doc:

My doctor wants to put me on blood pressure medicine, but I know my pressure only spikes at the office. It's normal at home. How can I prove this to my doctor?

Blood pressure rises and falls throughout the day and night depending on many factors, so it's not unusual for someone to measure high at the office and lower when at home or elsewhere, especially for patients who feel anxious about the idea of possibly being diagnosed with high blood pressure. Called "white coat hypertension," some patients experience elevated pressure only when they are at the doctor's office.

But, despite popular belief, white coat hypertension isn't benign. When Japanese researchers tracked the health outcomes of 128 people with white coat hypertension for eight years, as well as those of 649 people without the condition, the patients with white coat hypertension at the study's beginning were much more likely to develop full-blown hypertension within six years.[27]

To get a better picture of the rise and fall of your blood pressure, ask your health care provider to check your blood pressure over a 24-hour period. Ambulatory 24-hour blood pressure monitors look a lot like the heart rhythm monitors we use for irregular beat detection, but they record blood pressure instead. These monitors are covered by most insurers and give a wealth of information as to whether your blood pressure is truly normal during the entire day.

The monitor will automatically record your pressure every 15 to 30 minutes, providing 50 to 100 readings in all. The data from the device is then downloaded into software that your physician can analyze. It's thought that this type of monitoring is a much more accurate predictor of heart disease risk than the readings we take once a year at the office.

I check for what type of MTHFR gene is present. A defect, like the one I have, indicates the need for methylated B vitamins.

Lipoprotein-a. Lipoprotein-a or Lpa is an inherited form of the LDL cholesterol bound to a special protein. Much research has connected high levels of Lpa to early cardiovascular disease. This is a widely available blood test. I draw it on my patients if they have an abnormal calcium score or a thick carotid artery, as well as anyone with any sign of heart disease at a young age. High levels can be treated with niacin, hormone replacement, and vitamins. Most labs indicate a normal Lpa is under 30 mg/dl but I have seen readings reaching as high as 200 mg/dl. If you test high, consider it an opportunity to incorporate lifestyle changes that will lower the LDL cholesterol particle number a bit more and lower the Lpa level, too.

Fasting blood sugar, insulin, and A1c. Any standard blood panel will check your fasting blood sugar. Health care providers may not worry you until your blood sugar is in the diabetic range of more than 125 mg/dl, but studies suggest that a fasting blood sugar of less than 85 mg/dl is optimal. Each jump above 85 increases the risk of blood vessel injury. Blood sugar, however, only presents half of the equation because it is regulated by insulin. If the level of insulin is elevated, the pancreas is working "overtime" to maintain blood sugar and the arteries are at risk. If both the fasting blood sugar and the fasting insulin are normal, glucose metabolism is normal. I also often order a hemoglobin A1c to look at average blood sugar levels over a two- to three-month period. This is a sneaky way of checking for pathologic glycation—or sugar coating—of the hemoglobin molecule. It turns out elevated blood sugar levels not only coat the hemoglobin molecule, but they also coat the cholesterol particles, modifying them to become more dangerous.

Vitamin D. A low vitamin D level has been associated with high blood pressure, arterial damage, congestive heart failure, poor brain health, and other important problems. Normally vitamin D is obtained from sunlight and foods such as mushrooms and vitamin D–fortified foods, but even in sunny areas, most people test low. People with dark skin are especially at risk for vitamin D deficiency as the skin pigment blocks sunlight from making vitamin D in the skin. Ask your health care provider to check your level; you want your blood level of vitamin D to be over 30 ng/ml (nanograms per milliliter) and, optimally, 50 to 80 ng/ml.

Ferritin. Ferritin is a protein in the blood that binds to iron. If ferritin levels are high or low, that means the same is true of iron. Iron overload can oxidize cells in the arteries, leading to heart disease. It can also make the blood more prone to clotting. Iron overload in the organs can be checked by a simple ferritin test. Levels above 380 µg/l indicate iron excess. If you test high in ferritin, take care to avoid iron in vitamins and high-iron foods like red meat. Donating blood once a quarter, if possible, can lower your own iron levels while helping others at the same time.

Uric acid levels and GGT. These two simple and older blood examinations are coming back in use as they provide unique insight to the health of the cardiovascular system. Uric acid is produced from energy products like ATP (the energy used by cells), and an elevated level is linked to cardiovascular damage. GGT is a liver enzyme that may indicate an overall poor functioning of cell membranes in the liver and provide an insight to the overall health of your metabolism. Normal uric acid levels are 4 to 8 mg/dl and levels over 10 are concerning. Normal levels of GGT will fall below 50 IU/l (international units per liter), and levels over 100 IU/L are concerning for generalized cell membrane dysfunction.

Thyroid hormones. Many environmental toxins affect the thyroid gland, especially endocrine disruptors such as plastics. You'll learn more about those in Chapter 10. An advanced thyroid panel will include a bunch of designations that may look like a combination of shorthand and algebra: TSH, free T4, free T3, and the TPO antibodies. These are just abbreviations for different types of thyroid hormones and antibodies. What's important are your results. A normal result will vary depending on how the lab runs the test, but your readout will compare your result to the lab normal. The ideal TSH, to avoid subclinical hypothyroidism (underactive thyroid), is to have less than 2.5 mIU/l. A sign of overactive thyroid: undetectable TSH and elevated T4 and T3.

Sex hormones. If you are a man, make sure the lab measures total and free testosterone, DHEA, and estradiol levels. If you are a woman, learn the same labs along with progesterone levels.

Micronutrient testing. It is now possible to measure over 30 intracellular (inside of cells) vitamins, minerals, antioxidants, and amino acids. This test has only recently become available. With our unreliable lifestyles and food quality, it is very hard to know if cells are getting the nutrition they need. This blood test is covered by many insurance companies and can be very valuable to patients with serious diseases, including congestive heart failure, hypertension, and diabetes.

So that's a lot of blood work. The good news is that all but the last two are usually covered by insurance, and all can be completed with just one blood draw and one visit to your health care provider to go over your results. If you have limited insurance, then find a physician who offers a testing service called Health Diagnostic Laboratory Inc. (HDL Labs for short). These labs offer advanced testing and can give you the near-ultimate profile for the minimum cost, or at least this is what I've found in my clinic.

The Ultimate SHARK Detector: You

I know this may seem like a lot of information and tests, but keep in mind that heart disease is the most common cause of death and disability in the world. Don't allow this silent killer to cut your life short. Find it before it's too late.

Sure, you certainly can start on your holistic heart plan without having a single test done. I've found, however, that test results function a lot like truth serum. They strip away the denial that tells you, "Oh, one order of fries isn't going to kill me" and "I'll worry about my stress once things calm down." When you have heart disease, moderation can create moderate heart attacks and death. These tests motivate you to change quickly.

You can have all of these tests done in just one day, but you'll have to ask for them, and you might have to pay for some of them out of pocket. Since the average heart-clogging restaurant meal runs your family $50 or so, consider eating at home and using that money to get your heart checked instead.

Then, do everything you can to improve your scores. Add years to your heart. Don't take years away. Live to retire and watch your grandchildren grow. Have a full, vibrant old age.

Chapter 5

Your Whole Heart Ally

I encourage you to visit your health care provider *before* you start changing your lifestyle, and to follow up with him or her and stay in touch throughout your health journey. That's because your health care provider may very well be your most important ally when it comes to good heart health. Your health care provider may be a medical, osteopathic, or naturopathic doctor, nurse practitioner, or physician assistant.

Your health care provider knows you and your health history. As a result, your health care provider can help ensure that changes to your lifestyle don't interact with medicines you might be taking (and vice versa). As your lifestyle changes start to improve your heart health, your health care provider can help reduce your dosage of prescription medicines as needed. Your health care provider can also run various tests to help you see which changes are working and which are not.

Perhaps most important: Your health care provider can answer your questions, offer advice, and work with you to solve problems you might encounter. Ideally, your health care provider should be one of your most trusted sources of health information. He or she should be someone with a personality that not only puts you at ease, but allows you to feel comfortable asking questions, especially about recommendations you find unsettling.

But, if you are like many patients, this isn't the case. According to a survey conducted by General Electric in conjunction with the Cleveland Clinic, half of patients would rather do household chores than go to the doctor.[28] This concerns me.

It's unfortunate that so many health care professionals do not treat the whole patient. While they are quite knowledgeable about prescription medications, office procedures, and surgery, few know enough about nutrition and supplements to offer any useful advice. They weren't taught about either in medical school, and they haven't taken steps to learn more since. Sadly, some are more out of shape and overweight than the patients they are supposed to be helping.

One study done at UCLA found that health care providers fell short when it came to talking about dietary supplements.[29] The researchers analyzed transcripts of audio recordings from office visits to 102 primary care providers, checking to see how these health professionals covered five topic areas: the reason for taking the supplements, how to take them, their potential risks, their effectiveness, and their cost. I don't know about you, but those all seem like important pieces of information to me.

The researchers found that:

* Fewer than 25 percent of the five major topics were discussed during the office visits.

* All five topics were covered during discussions of only six of the 738 supplements.

* None of the five major topics was discussed for 281 of the supplements patients told their physicians they were taking.

When I hear such stories from patients about the health care providers they've seen who offered no support for their lifestyle changes and nutrition supplements, it saddens me.

I want to let you in on what might be the most important secret in this entire book: Not all health care providers rush their patients through an office visit like a shopper rushes through a discount store on Black Friday. Many of us care deeply for our patients. We enjoy spending time with them and we work hard to help them achieve healthy outcomes. We do our best to give our patients plenty of time and resources to bring up concerns and ask questions. We are never offended by questions. To the contrary: We wish patients would ask more of them. Rather than act annoyed when our patients bring up information they've read on the Internet or in magazines, we're delighted. That means our patients are being proactive about their health. Proactive patients tend to get and stay healthy. Apathetic patients? Not so much.

Your health care provider should *not* be someone you fear, someone you have a hard time understanding, or someone you want to avoid! And, I hope it goes without saying, your health care provider also should not seem rushed, as if he or she is not listening to your concerns.

This is why one of the most important changes you can make for your heart health may very well be this: Find a health care provider who helps you embark on a heart-healthy lifestyle and will support your efforts to be your best. How do you know if it's time to find a new provider? Try this: Make an appointment and bring this book with you. Mention your new lifestyle changes. Gauge the reaction. Hopefully your health care provider will respond by:

* Asking to read the book. If they want to buy their own copy, even better!
* Asking you what you thought of the book.
* Expressing an interest in integrative therapies and asking how you are doing with them.
* Exhibiting an open mind and a desire to learn more.
* Making a note to read about the topic.

If you get that reaction, you've probably found your health soul mate. On the other hand, if your provider merely mumbles something like "yeah, whatever, here's your prescription," it's probably time to enter the dating pool. Interview potential health care providers as you would interview a potential date. Ask them about their philosophy, roughly how much time they budget for sick and well visits, whether they prescribe supplements in lieu of (or in addition to) medications, and how they work to promote a healthy, active lifestyle. You should like the answers you hear to those questions. If you don't, you haven't found "The One." Hopefully you won't see two-liter bottles of soda and empty doughnut and candy boxes in the office . . . if you do, keep shopping!

A good relationship with your provider should feel not much different than the relationship you have with a trusted friend. You shouldn't feel as if you are being talked down to, manipulated, or ignored. You should feel seen and heard. Once you find an empathetic, knowledgeable, and dedicated health care provider, the rest is merely a matter of communication. The advice in the rest of this chapter will help you communicate effectively.

ASK YOUR HEALTH CARE PROVIDER TO WRITE THINGS DOWN

Many patients fail to follow doctor's orders not because they are rebels, but rather because they simply can't remember them. And many of us health care providers are so used to saying certain terms that we don't realize how confusing they sound to a patient's ears.

So don't just nod your head and pretend you understand. Don't assume you will remember everything your health care provider has told you, either. I frequently write lifestyle advice on a prescription pad and hand it to patients. Ask your health care provider to jot down:

* The correct spelling of over-the-counter medications or supplements he or she recommends, along with the dosage to take.

* URLs for websites where you can find more information.

* Books to read.

* Videos to watch.

Your health care provider also may have brochures that you can take with you that could be helpful, so ask for them.

TELL YOUR HEALTH CARE PROVIDER ALL OF YOUR SECRETS

According to the same General Electric survey I mentioned earlier, about 28 percent of patients sometimes lie or omit facts when talking to their health care providers.[30]

I suspect that number might be much higher, and I completely understand. Some health conditions are hard to talk about. On top of that, you might be forced to talk about embarrassing issues while you are only partially clothed. And if you don't have a good relationship with your health care provider, then you might just want to get the appointment over with as quickly as possible.

But holding back only hurts you. When we physicians don't know the full health picture, it's a lot harder for us to make an accurate diagnosis and to suggest an effective treatment.

So write down what you plan to tell your provider before you get to the office. Use the list to jog your memory. If you can't get the words out, allow your health care provider to read your list. One better: Ask a loved one to come with you, someone you trust to bring up issues that you might not feel comfortable talking about.

Frank's Journey to a Lasting Heart

After being prescribed his sixth new medication in 12 months, Frank was sick and tired of being sick and tired. He was a 70-year-old retired man with a belly a bit too round for optimal health. Because of the extra weight, he had developed high blood pressure, elevated blood sugar, and high triglyceride fats in the blood.

He felt overmedicated, so he did some research on the Internet and found a registry listing integrative health care providers. He began working with one nearby and changed his diet to organic foods and filtered water. He also started walking with a goal of 10,000 steps a day, sleeping at least seven hours a night, and using breathing exercises to reduce stress.

By the time he came to me, he had been able to get off of one prediabetic medication by making these lifestyle changes. I took a history from him and asked to see a list of everything he was taking. He showed me the prescription drugs and a bag with 12 supplements! He seemed tense as he handed them to me. I quickly browsed them and casually said things like, "Wow, what a great brand," or "This one will really help your blood pressure," or "I take the same thing," and so on. He stood and stared.

Further questioning revealed that I was actually the second cardiologist he had seen. Eight weeks earlier he had seen a highly regarded physician who laughed at him for being duped into taking the vitamins. When Frank asked that doctor what he thought about one of the vitamins, the doctor indicated that he hadn't the slightest idea how it worked, saying, "It can't be good if I've never heard of it."

Frank was turned off. That's when he sought me out. It turned out the supplement that had prompted the first heart specialist's laughter was alpha-lipoic acid, an antioxidant that has been shown in randomized scientific studies to prevent diabetic nerve damage just as well as any prescription medications. Needless to say, I got along great with Frank, earned his trust, and have worked with him now for four years. He is now down to two prescription medications for his blood pressure, has lost 18 pounds, and feels vibrant.

On your list, write down the following, all of which is helpful information for your health care provider:

* Your supplement list.

* Tests other health care providers have done.

* Prescribed medicines, whether you are taking them or not (and if you're not, why).

* Changes in your lifestyle (a new exercise plan, a new meditation class, etc.).

* Any sudden life stress, such as a job loss or a recent death in the family.

* Whether or not you are sticking to your diet or fitness plan.

LEARN AS MUCH AS YOU CAN

There are at least two types of patients: those who do their homework before they ever walk into the office and those who don't. The patients in the first category generally end up with better outcomes and that's often because they ask better questions. Rather than taking no for an answer, they are able to follow up with, "Well, I was reading about this treatment. Do you think it might work for me?" Very often, the answer might be yes.

In this book, I've tried to do most of this legwork for you. In the previous chapter, you learned about tests to suggest. In Part Two, you'll find dozens of lifestyle suggestions. Still, I recommend you read as much as you can. In the appendix of this book, I've listed dozens of resources. Consult them—and do so often. This will help you advocate most effectively for your health.

GUARD THIS RELATIONSHIP WITH YOUR LIFE

The relationship you have with your health care provider may very well be one of the most important relationships in your life. If you are with a dedicated health care provider who stays on top of health literature, you'll find that there's nothing you can bring up that causes your health care provider to seem put off. Much to the contrary, your health care provider will be able

Ask the Holistic Heart Doc:
How long should I stay in cardiac rehab?

If you have suffered a heart attack, had a heart stent inserted, or made it through bypass surgery, you'll be referred for cardiac rehabilitation. Don't skip these appointments. They literally could save your life. Patients in cardiac rehab programs have a 25 percent lower risk of death than patients who skip them, and they are also less likely to end up in the ER.

Your insurer will probably cover four to 12 weeks of one-hour sessions, three times a week, but don't stop there. You might have to pay a few dollars out of pocket for some sessions, but long-term rehab is well worth the cost. I have some patients who have been attending cardiac rehab for almost 20 years! They enjoy it that much. Social connectedness promotes wellness and survival, and cardiac rehabilitation often becomes a healthy club where dinner events, to talk about the pros and cons calmly, and in a way you can understand.

I don't think I can stress this any more strongly. If you are not in a comfortable relationship with your health care provider, it's time to break things off. Search for a new health care provider. And once you find a winner, hold up your end of the relationship. Ask questions. Listen with interest. Write things down as needed. If you don't feel comfortable with a recommendation, say so . . . doctor's orders!

award ceremonies, and general fun and laughter are encouraged. The sharing of experiences seems to raise the confidence, and maybe more than just the confidence, of participants in healthy lifestyle activities.

In particular, see if your community offers programs patterned after the work of Nathan Pritikin or Dr. Dean Ornish. These programs offer more hours a week of training with more emphasis on the low-fat, plant-based diets, mind/body stress management, and group sessions that make the work of these two pioneers shine bright. To get insurance coverage, ask your health care provider to write a referral. Patients of mine have attended these programs after I wrote a supportive letter, and go further faster than those in any other programs I have seen. One of my patients just came back from the Pritikin Center in Miami. She was beaming about her 12-pound weight loss and 30-point drop in cholesterol after just two weeks spent eating their plant-based diet.

Part Two

Whole Heart Prescriptions

If you read every page of Part One, then give yourself a big pat on the back. If I were the Wizard of Oz, I'd hand you a diploma for Integrative Cardiology because you now have a broader view of whole heart health than most health professionals do.

Now it's time to put your knowledge to practice. In the following pages, you'll find dozens of holistic heart practices. Every single one of them is powerful, proven by research, and road tested by myself and my patients. Which ones should you try first? How many do you need? The answers to those questions depend on your health and your motivation. The sicker you are, the more important it is to make big changes quickly—and the more motivated you'll feel to make them. Remember, the most impactful changes can be found in the earlier chapters; within each chapter, prescriptions are listed in order from easiest to implement to least.

No matter where you are in your health journey, pick the prescriptions that make the most sense to you and go at your own pace. Over time, as you incorporate more and more prescriptions, you'll start to feel younger, more energetic, and happier—and your heart will be healthier, too.

Chapter 6

Your Nutrition Rx

The Greek philosopher and physician Hippocrates said more than 2,000 years ago that food is medicine. After helping patient after patient prevent and reverse heart disease just by changing what they do and don't eat, I know that statement is completely accurate. It's my hope that, by the end of this chapter, you will as well.

More than two decades ago, Caldwell Esselstyn Jr., MD, of the Cleveland Clinic stumbled across a startling fact: Certain cultures around the world did not suffer from heart disease. He wanted to know why, so he began researching the eating habits of people in Papua New Guinea, rural China, central Africa, and the Tarahumara Indians of Mexico. He learned that these cultures consumed a plant-based diet free from meat, eggs, dairy, and added oils. He wondered: If Americans followed the same diet, would heart disease disappear?

He set out to find out. In the mid-1980s, he began recruiting heart disease patients. He ended up with men and women whose heart disease was so advanced that they were deemed too sick for bypass surgery. The results were startling. Of the patients who followed the diet for five years or longer, total cholesterol dropped almost 100 points (going from 246 mg/dl to 150 mg/dl), artery lesions shrank in size, and the progression of heart disease not only halted—it reversed itself. Esselstyn has stayed in touch with the participants ever since and those who stayed on the diet have not had a single additional heart attack, whereas those who regressed to their old eating habits did.[31]

I had the pleasure of lecturing with Dr. Esselstyn more than a dozen years ago and was completely taken by his confidence and the power of his scientific data. I read his papers and later his book describing his results. I believe in his approach so much that, with a few modifications, my own diet as well as many of my own food prescriptions are based on it. The point is this: The research is clear. The most powerful heart drug ever invented cannot be found at a pharmacy. Rather, it's sold at the grocery store or farmer's market, the real "farmacy."

Being mindful of what you put on and in your body is the most important step to preventing heart disease and ensuring total body wellness and vitality.

But you've heard at least some of it before. The problem with what you've probably heard, however, is this: Most health care providers (and even most cookbooks) don't give you the full story. Some of the foods you've been taught to sort into the "heart-healthy" category are anything but. Similarly, some other foods are so good for you that you really ought to think of them as medicine—but no one has bothered to tell you about them. And some other foods that you might be avoiding probably aren't as destructive to your health as you've been led to believe.

As one example, you've probably been told to eat five servings of fruits and vegetables a day. Well, guess what? That's probably only half of what you really ought to be consuming for optimal health.

Similarly, maybe you've been told that diet soda is better than regular or that skinless chicken breast is better than steak. You know what? They're all pretty bad for your heart.

I've read through all the studies and tried different approaches personally and with my patients, and I'm convinced that the best diet for optimal heart health is a low-fat, plant-based, vegan diet, the same diet that former president Bill Clinton followed after his heart scare. That's the diet I follow and that I prescribe for most of my patients. But I know that's not for everyone, or at least not right away. That's why I've provided you with some incremental steps and alternatives in the form of the prescriptions in this chapter. If you incorporate just one, you'll add life to your heart. And the more you do, the better you'll feel and the more you'll want to do. Even if you eat only one extra organic apple a day, you will have helped your heart.

To understand the importance of each prescription, you'll need a little nutritional 101.

HOW FOOD HEALS

What makes some foods heart healthy, but others heart harming? Let's take a journey through the human body, starting with the very first place your food lands: the GI tract.

Starting at our mouth, the GI system is a long tube and the cells that line it are supposed to be tightly bound one to another to keep undesirable wastes out of the bloodstream. Trillions of bacteria live here, in our GI tracts. We have so many bacteria in our guts that, if the stuff were scooped out and removed, we'd all lose about three pounds on the scale. These tiny little beings don't just take up space. They are very active. As churned-up slop makes its way out of the stomach and into the small and then large intestine, the bacteria feed on it. For the most part, this is helpful. By feeding on partially digested food, bacteria help to break down fiber and food. As they do so, they produce many beneficial byproducts, including health-promoting fatty acids and vitamins.

Eat heart-healthy plant-based foods, especially organic ones, and you'll nourish health-promoting bacteria that emit byproducts that turn down inflammation, neutralize toxins, and nourish cells and tissues. Eat heart-harming foods rich in chemicals, sugars, and other toxins, however, and you feed the bad guys. As these harmful bugs munch on the remnants of your lunch, they emit poisons and toxins. One of the toxins these bacteria produce is called *endotoxin,* and the immune system treats it as poison. When this toxin gets into the bloodstream, inflammation goes up.

When British researchers analyzed 40 different extracts made from various foods, they found that certain foods—especially animal products—contained high amounts of the very endotoxin that triggers health-harming inflammation in the body. Research has shown that cooking, boiling, and even treating these foods with acid does not prevent the inflammatory reaction they create.

Now, let's move a little farther along in the digestive journey and into the bloodstream. Here, the body works hard to keep levels of glucose (also called blood sugar) steady. If you consume heart-healthy foods, you help your body in this quest. Plant-based whole foods digest slowly, providing a slow, steady rise in blood sugar that the body is equipped to handle. Many heart-harming processed foods, on the other hand, digest quickly, dumping more sugar into the bloodstream than hormones and cells are capable of handling. If you eat blood sugar–spiking foods meal after meal, day after day, and week after week, you do much more than set the stage for diabetes; you also set it for heart disease.

In addition to blood sugar, heart-harming foods also flood the bloodstream with tiny globs of fat—carried by particles rich in triglycerides (fat). Think of these like a taxi carrying you through a busy downtown area, delivering you to your destination. Whenever you eat high-fat foods, your body converts the excess calories into these tiny packages of fat, and they float through the blood until they find a home, usually inside a fat cell. Continually overeat the wrong types of processed and animal-based junk foods and triglyceride levels remain elevated and stuff your muscle cells full of fat globules. Over time, this makes it harder for your body to control blood sugar and it also flames inflammation. In one study, people with the highest levels of these blood fats were four times more likely to develop heart disease and stroke than people with the lowest levels.[32]

Finally, certain foods truly act like medicine for your blood vessels. Healthy blood vessels are flexible, and widen to accommodate increased blood flow. Foods such as fruits (particularly pomegranates and grapes) and vegetables (particularly green leafy vegetables and beets), cacao chocolate, fish oil, teas, and soy all help arteries relax, driving down blood pressure and making it easier for the heart to pump blood. Other foods (especially those rich in sodium and certain types of fat) cause blood vessels to stiffen, squeezing them smaller to permit less blood to reach vital parts of the body. This can happen as soon as 30 minutes after a meal.[33]

So, I hope you can see, the overall prescription I hope you'll glean from this chapter is this: ***Consume more of the right foods (organic, single-ingredient, plant-based, whole foods) and fewer of the wrong ones (highly processed, high-fat, animal-laden dishes) and you'll help to protect your heart rather than speed its demise.***

Are you limited for the rest of your life to eating a raw sweet potato and steamed broccoli on a glass plate? Not at all! You'll be delighted to learn that you can improve your heart health right away—in the next 20 minutes—just by following the very first prescription in this chapter. And you can experience huge benefits by adding a few more.

Power Rx: Eat Leafy Greens to Lower Blood Pressure All Day Long

Nitrates are a class of drugs used to treat angina, or chest pain. They work by dilating the blood vessels and allowing more oxygen-rich blood to reach the heart. When you take a fast-acting form, you usually dissolve it under the tongue or spray it in the mouth—and the effect is near immediate. Most people experience relief of chest pressure or shortness of breath within five minutes.

Well, some foods contain a chemical similar to what's found in those prescription nitrates and almost as effective. While not a substitute for medications, arugula, lettuce, rhubarb, beets, pine nuts, kale, bok choy, cabbage, fennel, and spinach are all rich sources of nitrates, a form of nitrogen that they absorb from the soil. When we eat these foods, enzymes and bacteria in our mouths—and especially in the crevices on our tongues—convert those nitrates into nitrite.

When that nitrite gets to the stomach, acid reduces it to an important gas: nitric oxide. This simple chemical may very well be the most studied of recent years, and perhaps one of the most important. The scientist who described its functions earned a Nobel Prize in medicine. It makes arteries resist contraction, plaque, and blood coagulation, so strokes and heart attacks can't occur. It keeps arteries healthy, open, and free of clots.

Researchers at Queen Mary University of London recently found that those who consumed a nitrate-rich meal—such as a bowl of lettuce—experienced an 11.2-mmHg drop in blood pressure within just a few hours, a reduction that lasted all day long.[34] This is an important improvement in blood pressure that rivals the best results of powerful and widely prescribed drugs. It lowers the risk of stroke and heart attack substantially.

So go ahead and make yourself a salad, one that is rich in greens. Arugula happens to be the richest food source of nitrate, but other greens such as Swiss chard, kale, and spinach are great, too.

Rx at a Glance

To dose your blood vessels with nitric oxide:

* **Fill up on salad.** You do not need to be deprived or constantly hungry to be healthy and have a strong heart. I have worked with several finalists on *The Biggest Loser* show. They were all given the largest salad bowl you can imagine and were permitted to fill it as many times a day as they wanted. No, there was no meat, cheese, or eggs on the salad bar; only balsamic and red wine vinegar were used as dressings. Their salad fixings had so much bulk

Galen's Journey to a Lasting Heart

When Galen came to see me five years ago, he thought he was invincible. At the age of 54, he was running half and full marathons, a pursuit he thought of as an insurance policy for his heart. His complaint: fatigue. His race times were getting slower and slower.

Galen was thin, fit, and took no prescription drugs. Most people would take one look at him and think, "That's the last guy who will ever have a heart attack." I knew better.

When I examined him, I thought he looked healthy, but his electrocardiogram concerned me. The readout looked like his heart might not be getting all the oxygen it needed. So I asked him to get a coronary calcium CT scan (see page 57). Sure enough, he had heavy deposits of plaque in all three of his coronary arteries. I then had him complete a formal exercise stress test. He almost broke the treadmill . . . he could stay on so long at such a fast speed. He clearly did not need a heart catheterization.

Still I was concerned. We discussed his lifestyle, and I learned that he would often treat himself after training for an event by indulging in sweets, doughnuts, pizza, and fried foods. Was the junk food the cause of his fatigue and strange ECG? I decided to try an experiment, and I gave him the following prescription:

- Watch *Forks Over Knives,* a movie documentary detailing the health benefits of plant-based, whole food diets.
- Read *Prevent and Reverse Heart Disease* by Dr. Caldwell Esselstyn.

When Galen returned four weeks later, he bounced into the office with a smile and a handshake. He'd not only followed doctor's orders, he'd gone nearly the whole month without junk foods, processed foods, or animal products.

"I've never felt better," he told me. He had more energy, felt happier, and was running faster than he had before. His bowels were now regular and he was sleeping well, too. It has been five years and Galen's commitment to eating healthy foods has only increased. He has passed all subsequent stress tests, and I anticipate that he will never need a stent or a bypass operation.

and were so dense in nutrition that the participants were able to fill their stomach's capacity with a lot of nutrition and relatively few calories. Their waistlines and arteries benefited at the same time. Try my kale, arugula, and avocado salad (below).

* **Add greens to everything.** That includes soups, sandwiches, smoothies, and whatever else you can think of.

* **Eat more vegetables.** In addition to greens, many other vegetables are also rich in nitrates, especially celery and beets. A glass of beet juice a day may very well keep the blood pressure drugs away.

Natural Nitrate on a Plate

Heart-Healthy Dressing:
- 2 tablespoons balsamic vinegar
- 1 teaspoon lemon juice
- 1 teaspoon each of cayenne pepper, freshly ground black pepper, turmeric, and oregano
- 1 tablespoon Dijon mustard
- 2 tablespoons pomegranate juice

Salad:
- 4 cups chopped kale leaves
- 2 cups chopped arugula
- ½ cup halved cherry tomatoes
- ½ cup pine nuts and sesame seeds
- 1 ripe avocado, peeled, sliced into bite-size chunks

Toss in a large bowl. Add dressing to taste.

Power Rx: Add Spices to Everything

One of the easiest ways to protect your heart is also the tastiest. Many herbs and spices are medicine for the body. That's because they are concentrated from plants, so they contain the same protective chemicals that plants use to ward off pests and disease. When we consume these chemicals from the spices made from these plants, they protect the cells in our bodies from disease, too. Some of the heavy hitters include:

* **Garlic.** The allium in garlic has been shown to improve blood cholesterol, reduce blood pressure, and lower risk of developing heart disease.[35]

* **Turmeric.** The main ingredient in curry spice, turmeric is rich in curcumin, which has been shown to reduce cholesterol, triglycerides, and blood sugar. It also improves endothelial function.[36]

* **Ginger.** This natural anti-inflammatory herb has been shown to thin the blood and may also help reduce cholesterol.

* **Cinnamon.** This sweet spice is a natural antioxidant that may improve blood flow and help normalize blood sugar.[37]

* **Coriander.** In animals, this spice has been shown to lower blood cholesterol.[38]

Those are just a few of hundreds of healing spices. Others include cloves, allspice, nutmeg, oregano, rosemary, and many more.

Rx at a Glance

Use spices liberally, on everything you eat.

* **Sprinkle apple pie spice** (which contains cinnamon along with cloves, allspice, and nutmeg) on fruit, oatmeal, smoothies, and even your morning cup of joe.

* **Add Italian seasoning mix** (rich in several different antioxidant spices) onto salads, into soups, and onto potatoes and everything else that could benefit from some more flavor.

* **Embrace curry.** This may be one of the most powerfully healing spices around. In addition to traditional Indian and Thai curry dishes, you can sprinkle this spice on just about anything and end up with a delicious result.

Power Rx: Buy Organic

More than 400 chemicals are regularly used to kill weeds, insects, and other pests. Conventionally grown apples are sprayed as many as 16 times with 36 different pesticides! Conventional produce may have 90 times the pesticide content of organic produce.

When researchers from Uppsala University in Sweden took blood samples from more than a thousand elderly Swedes, analyzed them for pesticides, and compared those levels to existing heart disease, they arrived at rather disturbing findings. People with more pesticides in their blood were at a higher risk for clogged arteries, and this was true regardless of their age, weight, blood pressure, and other health habits.[39]

In addition to directly affecting your heart health for the worse, ingesting pesticides may indirectly harm health by causing vitamin D deficiency.[40]

But there are several more compelling reasons to avoid pesticides: Organic produce is richer in heart-healthy phytonutrients. University of California at Davis researchers have found that organic tomatoes are richer in flavonoids than conventionally grown tomatoes. One possible reason why: Flavonoids help ward off pests, so tomatoes not treated with pesticides tend to naturally make more of the stuff.[41]

Rx at a Glance

Sadly, the very foods most likely to contain pesticides are the very ones you should be eating for good health: fruits and vegetables. When buying them, use this advice:

* **Eat a variety.** The more different kinds of fruits and vegetables you eat, the lower your exposure to any one pesticide.

* **Thoroughly wash all the produce you buy.**

* **Look for the NutriClean program seal** that some markets use to certify that their produce contains no detectable levels of pesticides.

* **If you can't afford to go 100 percent organic, at least do it for the most important foods.** According to the Environmental Working Group, the foods most likely to contain dangerous pesticide residues are apples, strawberries, grapes, celery, cherry tomatoes, cucumbers, hot peppers, nectarines, peaches, potatoes, spinach, sweet bell peppers, kale and collard greens, and summer squash. The foods least likely to contain residues and safest to buy conventionally grown? Asparagus, avocados, cabbage, cantaloupe, eggplant, grapefruit, kiwi, mushrooms, onions, pineapples, sweet peas, and sweet potatoes.

Power Rx: Drink More Tea

Unlike soft drinks, tea actually comes from a plant. As a result, it's a rich source of plant substances—called flavonoids—that help neutralize oxidation in the body. Green tea, in fact, is the best food source of a particular type of flavonoid called catechins. These substances protect our cells much like a premium gas additive keeps your car engine humming. And test tube studies show that catechins are more powerful than vitamins C, E, and other antioxidants.

Green, black, and oolong teas all help reduce heart disease in several ways, including by:

* Halting the oxidation of LDL cholesterol.

* Improving cholesterol and triglyceride levels.

* Blocking dietary cholesterol from being absorbed into the bloodstream.

* Regulating levels of blood sugar.

* Soothing inflammation.

It's no wonder that researchers from the Netherlands found that people who drank six cups of tea per day were 36 percent less likely to develop heart disease than people who drank one cup or fewer daily,[42] and why researchers have also found that countries that consumed the most tea had the lowest incidences of type 2 diabetes.[43]

Rx at a Glance

To make the most of tea, use this advice:

* **Drink one more cup of tea daily.** Every cup of tea you drink benefits your heart, so start with whatever amount is realistic for you. If you drink no tea, then one cup a day is a good goal. If you already drink some tea, then aim for three cups a day, having one with each meal. If you are already drinking three, then feel free to go for the full six by making tea one of your go-to beverages. If I am walking out the door with a hot mug in my hand, it will usually be full of green tea, often with a splash of rice milk.

* **Let your tea steep for 3 to 5 minutes.** This will boost the amount of catechins.

* **Drink unsweetened tea.** If you don't enjoy the plain flavor, jazz it up with lemon, lime, mint, or orange.

* **Drink fresh-brewed tea if you can.** Bottled and instant powdered teas contain fewer catechins, but these are still one huge step better than a sugar-sweetened beverage.

* **When dining out, ask for unsweetened iced tea.** It's a great option that most restaurants—and even some fast food establishments—offer.

Power Rx: Break Up with Soda and Other Sweetened Beverages

So perhaps you read the prescription about tea and you are sitting there thinking, "How can I fit in that much tea drinking?"

Here's how: Swap tea for other beverages, especially sugar-sweetened ones like soda.

Not only will you avoid between 130 and 190 calories per can, you'll also make dramatic strides toward siphoning one of the biggest heart killers out of your diet: sugar.

The average person in the United States and Canada ingests about 150 pounds of sugar (dry weight) a year. Think about a 50-pound bag of play sand you might buy to fill a sandbox and multiply by three. That would be quite a pile. In fact, food expert Jamie Oliver, famous for his *Food Revolution* TV series, made the point of this excessive consumption by dumping an oversized wheelbarrow full of sugar on stage.

One of the strongest concerns regarding sugar consumption and heart disease has been sugar-sweetened beverages like soda, vitamin waters, energy drinks, and even juices. Just one can of one of these beverages contains 10 to 12 teaspoons of sugar. Those with healthy-looking labels can have twice as much sugar.

Often referred to by health professionals as "liquid Satans," these sources of calories are handled differently by your body's appetite centers than solid food. These liquid calories don't seem to trigger the brain to curb your appetite. For example, when study participants consume 200 calories or so from a liquid an hour before a meal, they tend to eat a lot more during that meal than people who consumed the same number of calories from a solid food such as two pieces of fruit.[44] Liquid sugary calories like sodas just do not curb our hunger, and we eat more and get fatter and more inflamed as a result.

But these beverages also affect your heart. An amazing 180,000 people die each year, worldwide, due to the consumption of sugary drinks, and about 45,000 of those deaths are from heart attacks.[45] Heart disease might set in because people who drink many soft drinks tend to gain weight, become diabetic, and suffer premature heart blockages. But there are other mechanisms. Soft drinks elevate blood sugars, which, as I mentioned in Chapter 2, coat proteins and fats, rendering them into a harmful form that damages your arteries. An example of this process is the creation of advanced glycation end products or AGEs that prematurely age the heart and vessels. Another is the coating of cholesterol with sugar-coated LDL cholesterol, which is recognized as foreign by arteries and is taken up to create artery plaques.

Sugar-sweetened beverages can also erode heart health in another sneakier way: by creating a petri-dish-like environment in your mouth. Poor oral health—particularly of the gums—can lead to heart disease, and inflammation may be the common thread. Constantly bathing your teeth and gums with sugar might cause the proliferation of certain types of bacteria that are known to promote inflammation throughout the body, erode your tooth enamel, and rob your saliva's ability to convert certain vegetables into healthy nitrates.

No matter the mechanism, the end result is clear: heart disease. For more than two decades Harvard researchers have been studying more than 40,000 physicians and 88,000 nurses, asking them to keep diaries about their food and beverage intakes. If you are a soda lover, their results will break your heart.

Women who consumed more than two servings of a sugary beverage a day were 40 percent more likely to develop heart disease than women who drank fewer.

The men who drank the most sodas were 20 percent more likely to have a heart attack than those who drank the least.[46]

Just one sugary beverage a day boosted the risk of heart disease by 19 percent.[47]

And switching from a sugary drink to a diet drink is not a solution. Although artificial sweeteners are still allowed by our government agencies, there are more reports of adverse reactions to artificial sweeteners every year than any other food type. For your brain, for your heart, skip the yellow, blue, and pink packets of artificial sugars and the diet beverages that contain them.

Rx at a Glance

Clearly, drinking Dr Pepper and other sugary, sweet items is a good way to earn yourself an appointment with a cardiologist . . . or even a cardiac surgeon. Here's my advice:

* **Give up soda.** That's right. We're talking zero tolerance. Moderation maims. If you drink several of these a day, be realistic. Perhaps you swap one of those beverages for an iced tea or a seltzer. Or maybe you water your soda down, mixing half a glass of seltzer in with the soft drink. Over time, drink less and less soda until you get to zero. (If you see your health care provider drinking these, help him or her break the habit by sharing this information.)

* **Wean off fruit juice, too.** A glass of commercially prepared OJ has just as much sugar (in some cases even a little more) as your typical soft drink.

* **Make tea and water your beverage staples.** Consume eight glasses a day of tea and water. Several times a day, I like to have a large glass of room-temperature water with a slice of lemon, a practice going back thousands of years in the Indian Ayurvedic tradition. At least start the morning that way; try it and see what you think.

Power Rx: Enjoy Coffee in Moderation

For many years people at risk for developing heart disease were told to shun coffee. Actually, without the cream and artificial sweeteners, coffee is surprisingly healthy for most people, and, despite the caffeine it contains, a cup of dark roasted java may actually lower blood pressure rather than raise it. Its polyphenols (plant chemicals that protect against disease) might also help, too.

So there's no reason to stop drinking coffee if you love it, but you do want to keep your habit in check. Of course, if coffee gives you racing heartbeats or jitteriness, listen to your body and skip it.

Rx at a Glance

To enjoy your morning joe and reap good health, do the following:

* **Hold yourself to no more than four cups a day.** A recent study found that drinking more than four eight-ounce cups of coffee a day was associated with a shorter life span, so enjoy your java but limit it to reasonable amounts.[48]

* **Watch what you add to your coffee.** Your coffee might be heart healthy, but the fatty milk, sugar, syrups, and colorful packets of artificial sweeteners are not. If you don't like black coffee, consider trying a product called Dynamic Greens. It contains organic greens, fruits, and superfoods like goji berry, chlorella, and pomegranate extracts. I add it to my morning coffee and it makes the coffee taste like a mug of hot chocolate.

Power Rx: Eat More Plants (at Least Five Servings a Day)

There is one thing that just about every nutrition expert in the country agrees on: Plants are good for us. Whether it's a tomato or a butter bean or an onion, it's good for you. No one ever got sick from too many vegetables in their diet.

Nearly everything you could possibly buy in the produce section of your grocery store is true medicine to the body. Plant foods are rich in vitamins, minerals, fiber, and special compounds called phytonutrients (pronounced "fight-o-nutrients"), all of which are good for the heart. Think about phytonutrients as fighting for your health. Here are just a few examples:

* **Asparagus, bell peppers, and bok choy** are rich sources of B vitamins, especially B_6, which helps lower homocysteine (an amino acid linked to heart disease) and C-reactive protein (a marker of inflammation).

* **Carrots and tomatoes** (as well as the fruits oranges and bananas) are rich in carotenoids including lycopene, an important type of antioxidant.

* **Garlic, onions, and leeks** all contain sulfur, which is thought to help lower levels of blood cholesterol and improve methylation.

* **Beets are high in betaine,** another natural ingredient that spins the homocysteine cycle faster and promotes lower blood pressure and total body health.

It's no wonder that Harvard's Nurses' Health Study and Health Professionals Follow-Up Study—two of the largest and longest-running studies ever done—found that people who eat more fruits and vegetables have a lower risk of developing heart disease. People who ate 8 or more servings were 30 percent less likely to have a heart attack or stroke than people who consumed 1½ servings or fewer.[49] Even 1 serving a day trumps zero.

Other research has shown that plant-rich diets can drop systolic blood pressure (the upper number of a blood pressure reading) by about 11 mmHg and diastolic blood pressure (the lower number) by almost 6 mmHg. That's as effective as blood pressure–lowering medications. A recent Swedish study found that people who consume five or more servings of produce a day lived an average of three years longer than people who consumed none.[50]

And they've also been shown to prevent cancer and diabetes, improve GI health, and protect your eyes, among many, many other benefits.

Even if you don't give up meat, dairy, or processed foods, more servings of plants in your diet will improve your heart health. I call it the P/A ratio: Increase your consumption of plants (P) and decrease your consumption of animals (A) and your health will improve.

Try to eat at least five servings a day, but 10 would be much better. That's about one to two pounds a day of greens, beans, mushrooms, peppers, and so on.

How much do you think the average person is eating? Go ahead and take a stab at a number. Seven servings? Five? Four?

Try three.

And one, two, or often three of those servings come in the form of ketchup, fries, chips, and various potato products.

You probably don't need me to tell you that this just isn't a good thing.

Rx at a Glance

If you are like most people, you probably aren't anywhere close to the minimum serving of five plant foods a day. Here's some advice that will help you get there:

* **Eat one more serving of fruits and vegetables than you had yesterday.** Keep this up for a week. Next week, add another serving. Keep doing this until you've surpassed five and, ideally, keep going until you've hit somewhere between eight and 12 servings. Keep a log on your calendar or smartphone. Treat yourself to new walking shoes when you hit 10.

Ask the Holistic Heart Doc:

I've heard alcohol is good for heart health. What types of alcohol are best? And how much should I drink?

You've heard correctly: Alcohol does seem to promote heart health. An analysis of 84 different studies on the effects of alcohol on heart health pooled the data gathered from more than two million men and women over 11 years. Compared to people who didn't drink at all, moderate drinkers had a 25 percent lower risk of being diagnosed with heart disease and a 25 percent lower risk of dying from a heart attack. They also had a 13 percent lower risk of dying from any cause, including cancer.[51]

How does alcohol heal your heart? No one knows for sure. It's possible that antioxidant plant chemicals called flavonoids—especially from the grapes used to make red wine—help protect the blood vessels from damage. It's also possible, however, that moderate drinkers are also just healthier. People who drink moderately also tend to exercise and eat a diet rich in fruits and vegetables.

But there are some drawbacks. Some people are sensitive to alcohol and can easily become addicted to it. Too much alcohol is also toxic, so you don't want to overdo it. Plus alcohol and dangerous machinery don't mix. Never attempt to operate a motor vehicle, use a weed whacker or some other sharp bladed power tool, or handle a gun after you've been drinking.

My recommendation: Alcohol is optional. If you enjoy it, then drink moderately, no more than one or two drinks a day for men and one drink a day for women. One drink equals a 12-ounce beer, 4 ounces of wine, 1.5 ounces of 80-proof spirits, or 1 ounce of 100-proof spirits.

* **Definitely eat more salads.** Top everything with salsa, the fresher the better. Pack your soups full of veggies and dark leafy greens. Have one to two servings in

your morning smoothie. Top every single sandwich with vegetables or make it a lettuce wrap. Add veggies to every dish you make, and make some of them raw. For lunch, have a salad with a side of veggie soup and a piece of fruit.

* **Add one or two servings with dinner.** Make dinner rich with vegetables known to promote health and reduce cancer risk such as these big heart defenders: dark leafy greens (lettuce, spinach, Swiss chard, mustard greens), cruciferous vegetables (broccoli, cauliflower, cabbage, Brussels sprouts, bok choy, kale, wasabi), or citrus (oranges, lemons, limes, grapefruit). A great goal: Half your dinner plate should be fruits and vegetables.

* **Have them on hand.** You'll be a lot more likely to eat an apple if you have apples in your fridge. Here's another secret: Make sure they are easy to eat. If you have a whole pineapple sitting on your counter, you might eat it. But if you spend one day a week prepping fruits like melons and pineapple for the week to come, you can go from might to definitely will pretty quickly. The same is true for veggies. Spend a day chopping and storing onions, peppers, celery, broccoli, and other veggies. Keep easy-to-grab lettuce on hand, too.

* **Consume some of them raw and sprouted.** Cooking can reduce and, in some cases, destroy the healing properties in plants, so include a mix of raw plant foods (such as salads) as well as sprouted plants (such as broccoli sprouts, sprouted legumes, and sprouted grains), as these are often more concentrated in healing nutrients than their unsprouted cousins.

* **Go vegan.** One of the side benefits of forgoing meat, fish, dairy, and eggs is this: You'll automatically end

up filling up on fruits and veggies. Websites like www.pcrm.org offer free, simple 21-day plans to help you go vegan.

Power Rx: Study Food Labels Like Jane Goodall Studies Chimps

As you'll soon learn, processed foods come packaged with a number of heart-agers. Whether it's the high animal fat content, the excess salt inside of most canned foods, the plastic residues that linger on shrink-wrapped fare, or the toxins that literally have been cooked into certain products, many of them are better left on the shelf.

But let's face it: Sometimes we don't have a choice. A packaged convenience food might be our only hope at getting dinner onto the table rather than running out for fast food.

Avoiding harmful additives doesn't mean you can't ever eat foods from a box or a container, and it doesn't mean you must pay more for good health, either. On my trip to the grocery store not long ago, two brands of ketchup were side by side. One was from a famous producer; the other was private-labeled and marked "organic." The prices were within pennies of each other. The famous label had HFCS (high fructose corn syrup) as the third ingredient and corn syrup (both likely GMO products) as the fourth. The other brand had organic sugar as the third ingredient (non-GMO by definition) and 20 percent fewer calories from carbohydrates. The organic version also had less salt per serving. Is there any question which brand I purchased and which you should, too?

Rx at a Glance

Always check the list of ingredients. Always. Always. Always. And use these guidelines:

* **If sugar is one of the first ingredients or if high fructose corn syrup is listed, skip it.** Keep in mind that sugar has many aliases: dextrin, dextrose, glucose, honey, maltodextrin, malt syrup, maltose, saccharose, sorghum, sucrose, and any ingredient that includes the word "syrup."

* **If you see the words "partially hydrogenated," skip it.** Do this even if the food contains a claim on the front of the package: "Contains zero trans fat." This claim is misleading. The FDA currently allows companies to label foods with 0.5 gram or less trans fat per serving as "trans-fat free," even if they have 0.45 gram. In other words, on the label they round a 0.49-gram serving of trans fat down to zero rather than up to 1 gram. So if you had four processed items and a piece of meat during the day, your trans fat intake could be 2 to 3 grams, which is way in excess of desirable levels. (In other countries, such as Canada, the labeling laws are stricter. Companies can only round to zero if the food contains less than 0.049 gram. Otherwise, small amounts of trans fats are rounded down to 0.1 gram, which at least allows consumers to know that the food is not in fact "free" of trans fats, but contains small amounts.)

* **Don't buy foods with the following harmful additives:** aspartame, butylated hydroxyanisole (BHA), butylated hydroxytoluene (BHT), saccharin, sodium nitrite, sodium sulfite, or monosodium glutamate (MSG).

Power Rx: Skip Foods Made in Plants

I've told you about the healing power of plants. The opposite is true for most of the foods that have been manufactured inside of a plant. Processed foods—the foods that you find inside a box, bag, or plastic container—are much more likely to be inflammatory than a meal made from whole food ingredients.

That's because most processed foods contain one or more of the following additives:

Sugar. The American Heart Association recommends that no one consume more than 100 calories (or 6 to 9 teaspoons) of added sugar per day. Yet most people consume 18 to 23 teaspoons of the white stuff daily, according to the U.S. government's National Health and Nutrition Examination Survey, and a huge number of people consume more than one-third of their total calories from sugar. Much of that sugar comes from a beverage I've already warned you about: soft drinks. Just one 20-ounce bottle of soda contains 16 teaspoons of sugar! The rest, however, is stealthily packed into an array of packaged foods. Bread? Yep, it's in there. Crackers? There's sugar in those, too. It's even in some brands of frozen shrimp and tomato sauce.

High fructose corn syrup. Similar to sugar, you'll also find this additive in most processed foods—even ones that don't seem sweet. In one study, researchers asked study participants to go on what, for me, would have been a sugar binge, but what for many people is culinary business as usual. The study participants consumed one-quarter of their total calories from either HFCS or glucose (also a form of sugar). Within just two weeks, those on the HFCS-rich diet experienced spikes in blood concentrations of the harmful LDL cholesterol, triglycerides, and apolipoprotein B (a blood protein that contributes to clogged arteries and heart disease). Consumption of the same amount of glucose (another form of sugar) did not have the same effect.[52]

Is sugar worse? Is HFCS worse? That's up for debate. My take is this: No sweetener—whether it is made from corn, cane, or something else—will ever fall in the same sentence as "health food." Should you eat less sugar? Clearly the answer is yes. Should you drink fewer sweetened beverages? Again, the overwhelming response is yes. If you want to live a long and full life, minimize all sweeteners, including HFCS.

Partially hydrogenated vegetable oils. Also called trans fats, these fats are the worst types of fat you can consume. They come from two sources. Trans fats occur naturally in animal products such as meat. They are also made by the food industry by adding hydrogen to vegetable oil, thus the word "hydrogenated" in their name. This process makes the oil less likely to spoil, more like animal fats, and it's what allows so many foods to remain on a grocery shelf or in your pantry for years without growing mold or developing a not-so-appetizing odor.

The problem is that these fats raise levels of the LDL cholesterol and drop levels of the HDL, and Harvard research has linked them to an increased risk of heart attack.[53] These fats also promote inflammation, as well as hinder the response of endothelial cells that line your blood vessels. They also trigger insulin resistance.

Thankfully, many foods are now labeled trans-fat free, so people are consuming fewer and fewer of these harmful fats. Still, as you learned from the Power Rx on page 100, companies are allowed to label products trans-fat free if they have less than 0.5 gram of trans fats per serving.

Plastic. Bisphenol A (BPA) is a chemical used to make certain plastics, such as the thin sheet of plastic that coats many types of food containers. These chemicals can leak into the food. That's not good as dozens of studies have linked BPA to all sorts of health woes, including heart problems. You'll learn more about this dangerous toxin in Chapter 10.

Sodium. Sodium raises blood pressure in susceptible people, and more than 75 percent of the sodium most people consume comes from processed and restaurant foods. Very little of it actually comes from the saltshaker. Store-bought and restaurant-served bread has become the number one source of dietary sodium, even if you can't taste it.

Genetically modified ingredients. Genetically modified organisms (GMOs) were introduced into foods in 1994 with a delayed-ripening tomato called the Flavr Savr. Basically researchers altered the DNA of the tomato, turning off the genes that caused fast ripening and allowing tomatoes to last longer. Now most varieties of soy, corn, canola, cottonseed, and sugar contain GMOs. GMO salmon has also been approved. GMOs have been used to grow plants faster, resist pathogens, and produce extra nutrients. This may sound like a good plan, but it is really alarming on several levels. For one, a field of GMO wheat (or any other GMO crop) can contaminate other fields by blowing seeds, contaminating our food supply. Here's more. When a pest tries to eat GMO plants, the poison in the plant's DNA travels to the stomach of the pest, splitting it open and killing it. These poisons might not be strong enough to kill bigger animals like humans, but they still may harm us. Studies show that the ingestion of these foods raises markers of inflammation.[54] Although the effects of GMO foods on humans are not completely known, there is a growing movement in the United States to limit or label GMO foods, as new concerns have been raised about a possible relationship to the increasing frequency of food allergies and low vitamin D levels. Though more research is needed, it's of interest that 27 countries have entirely banned GMO food production and another 61 require all food items produced with GMO foods be labeled as such.

Rx at a Glance

Reading labels is so important and, if you took the previous prescription to heart, then you're already doing that. Still, for many people, much of what they insert into their mouths is not from a plant, but rather is made in a plant. If that's the case with you, then take baby steps. The biggest gift you can give yourself and your family is to become mindful of what you eat and demand safety and quality. Think about what you consume day in and day out. Jot down a list of typical fare that is made in a plant. Then see if you can make some small compromises. Here are some ideas:

* **If you must have chips, pair them with a plant.** For instance, dip snack chips in homemade low-fat

hummus or fresh salsa. The healthy dips will help to fill you up so you naturally consume fewer chips. Over time, mix in carrot or celery sticks for some of the chips. Eventually wean off the chips altogether.

* **Make a rule that no sandwich can pass your lips unless it contains at least some vegetables.** Make up to half of the sandwich contents lettuce, tomatoes, or avocado slices.

* **Once a week, spend time prepping whole foods for the week to come.** Cook up a big batch of wild rice. Chop up a bunch of fruit. Chop celery, peppers, and other veggies so you can easily toss them into various dishes. The more plants you have in the fridge that are easy to access, the less likely it will be that you end up eating something that was made in a plant.

* **Learn how to make some dishes from scratch.** For instance, you might want to impress your friends with homemade tomato sauce rather than using a store-bought variety.

Power Rx: Drive Past the Drive-Thru

Not long ago, Dr. Robert Vogel and his colleagues at the University of Maryland asked 10 healthy hospital employees—none of whom had heart disease—to consume 900 calories, 50 grams of fat, and 255 milligrams of cholesterol for breakfast, in the form of a Mc-Donald's Egg McMuffin and two hash browns.

It makes my heart hurt just thinking about it.

The employees chowed down. Then the researchers measured blood vessel activity every hour for several hours. As we learned earlier, normally when you compress and then release a blood vessel, blood flow increases above normal for a few minutes. But the volunteers who ate Egg McMuffins didn't experience this healthy reaction. It was quite the opposite. When the researchers pressed and then released their arms, there was a dramatic reduction in blood flow. Compared to volunteers who'd consumed a non-fat breakfast consisting of cereal, non-fat milk, and OJ, the McMuffin eaters had arteries that behaved as if a dose of poison had just been injected.[55] It took five hours for their arteries to recover!

And these were young, healthy volunteers.

Several other investigators have repeated, replicated, and expanded on the experiment. They've found that many different types of fast food raise markers of inflammation throughout the body, particularly attacking the blood vessels, the brain, the lungs, and the GI tract.

And these foods do this within minutes of your eating them.

That's because gas stations, fast food restaurants, and other grab-and-go fare purveyors tend to serve up the worst of the worst foods: sandwiches made from processed lunch meats, hot dogs, greasy burgers, fried food, soft drinks, and many options that aren't even truly food but rather a chemical health enemy (more about this very soon).

Sadly, there are actually 27 U.S. hospitals with McDonald's in their lobbies, and many more with Wendy's, Burger Kings, and other chains. Patients and their families are eating there and getting sicker . . . not healthier! That is blatantly absurd and embarrassing to the medical community. At one of the hospitals where I see patients, we had a national ice cream chain move into the hospital lobby a few years back. While I understand the ritual of an ice cream cone after a Little League game (although a crisp apple is healthier), watching visitors walk through the halls of the hospital with the double scoop special made my blood boil. This and other fast meals and snacks injure artery linings and cause a reduction in blood flow. What kind of message were we sending to the public and patients? I wrote letters and blogs to the administration, and after a few years the chain packed up and moved out. Common sense won out over cents! It was replaced by a gourmet grocer that sells Mediterranean-style foods, fresh vegetable sushi, and salads. One victory for the cardiologist, the visitors, and the patients!

Most fast food places, however, are not serving the healthy fare that we now have in the lobby of my hospital. Trying to find a healthful meal at fast food restaurants and gas stations can be like trying to find the one person at JFK Airport who isn't in a hurry. Even the so-called "healthy" fare—such as the fruit smoothies and the salads—are often not healthy at all. The chopped chicken salad at one fast food chain has more calories (640) and fat (46 grams) than many burger and fry combos! And the fruit smoothies offered at one chain contain sugar as the third ingredient. In other words, a huge portion of that cup is not fruit or fruit juice. It's sugar, and these smoothies only have 2 fewer grams of sugar than your typical Mountain Dew. The worst drink offender of all brought to us by food corporations? The Baskin-Robbins large Heath Bar shake. It may be just what you crave on a hot summer day, but this will add an amazing 2,310 calories to your waistline, 108 grams of fat (more than half of it saturated), and a grotesque 66 teaspoons of sugar. If you just cannot resist it, I advise either splitting it with 20 of your best friends or tasting it outside of an emergency room entrance, just in case.

Some of these chains have recently announced plans to increase fruit and vegetable options. I can only hope the changes will be substantial because, as of this writing, nearly everything sold at these places is rich in these heart-harming ingredients:

Sugar, fat, and salt. Perhaps you have read *The End of Overeating* by David Kessler, the former head of the Food & Drug Administration. Or maybe you've checked out the more recent *Salt Sugar Fat* by reporter Michael Moss. If you have, then you have begun to understand how the food industry has leaned on food scientists and chemists to create foods that are not only addictive, but also deadly. When we start eating foods that are high in fat, salt, and sugar, we just can't stop. That's why it's so hard to eat only a handful of potato chips. Food scientists know our weakness and have engineered these foods so they are irresistible, and it's nearly impossible to stop at just one.

It is not an accident that the average person is eating three to four times more cheese annually than several decades ago. Cheese sells food items, and many people eat it with every meal even though it is usually very high in saturated fat and salt and never has fiber or micronutrients. Say "cheese" at a photo shoot, but not at all your meals. Your body will smile bigger.

Corn. If left to their own preferences, cows would consume grass, vegetables, legumes, and whatever else they found as they wandered through a pasture. This type of a diet provides cows with antioxidants and minerals, keeping them—and the meat inside their bodies—healthy and high in omega-3 fatty acids.

In modern beef production practices, however, cows are not allowed to graze. Instead they are confined to tiny feedlots and fed corn and other grains that they normally would not eat. These foods increase inflammation inside the cows' bodies, creating pro-inflammatory nutrients that are stored in the meat that we eventually eat. Meat from corn-fed cows is lower in natural antioxidant nutrients and enzymes and much higher in a type of fat (omega-6 fatty acids) that tends to turn on inflammation throughout our bodies and lower in other types of fat (omega-3 fatty acids) known to cool inflammation. Beef from corn-fed cattle is also more likely to boost cholesterol levels than beef from grass-fed animals. Furthermore, the corn fed to most livestock is GMO corn and ends up in the bodies of people eating their flesh.

Hormones and antibiotics. These fast food meats also tend to come from animals that were injected with antibiotics and hormones. The antibiotics in the meat enter our bodies and alter the balance of good and bad bacteria that fill our bowels. It is estimated that about 85 percent of the bacteria in our colon are helpful and the remainder may contribute to disease. The overuse of antibiotics wipes out members of the healthy bacterial communities, allowing disease-causing bacteria to proliferate. The hormones in the meat lead to weight gain, diabetes, and perhaps many other chronic illnesses.

Fake food. Much of what you buy from fast food establishments isn't what it seems. The Cleveland Clinic pathology department recently collected eight different brands of fast food hamburgers from chains around the area (since they, sadly, have a McDonald's in their lobby, they only had to drive to get the other seven). The pathologists basically did an autopsy on the hamburgers, looking at them under the microscope and adding stains to examine what was in these "food" items. On average, the amount of beef that was measured in the burgers was 12 percent. The rest? Bacteria, parasites, non-meat animal parts, and even sawdust.[56] It's no wonder this toxic combination leads the body to view it as a foreign invader. When you eat non-food foods, that's exactly what happens. The body treats them like poison, and inflammation follows meal after meal. Another study did a similar autopsy on chicken nuggets. Steven Bigler, a pathologist at Baptist Health Systems in Jackson, Mississippi, stained, sliced, and analyzed the meat under a microscope, finding that it wasn't meat at all but rather "an artificial mixture of chicken parts." These doctors found that over half of the nugget was not meat but nerves, skin, blood vessels, and bone fragments.[57]

Endotoxin. I mentioned this bacterial toxin in the beginning of this chapter. What do you think happens after you eat an Egg McMuffin and hash browns or other types of fast food like them? It feeds the bacteria that produce endotoxin, and endotoxin is released into the bloodstream at levels far above baseline for several hours. Consider that 70 percent of the immune system is situated in and just around the gut. That means that inflammation-triggering white blood cells are right there, on the ready, as soon as endotoxin comes in. End result: sudden inflammation. A war of survival is activated after every bite from the white bag.

But here's more. These foods don't just nourish the bad bacteria in your gut and cause them to produce toxins, the foods themselves actually contain these toxins! One fast food quarter pounder may contain 100 million dead bacteria, give or take. And while the cooking might kill the bacteria, it doesn't remove the endotoxin.

Inside every artery is the endothelium. Its job is to keep arteries wide open, free of clots, and provide maximal blood flow to important organs. Researchers have shown that within just 60 minutes of eating a breakfast sausage sandwich and hash browns, the endothelium malfunctions. It behaves as if it's sick, leading to artery constriction. The same thing happens in airways, so take note if you have asthma. This goes on for five to six hours. What this means is blood vessels are less able to accommodate blood flow, are more prone to clotting, and get damaged. Do this to your arteries every day, and they harden and narrow.

Rx at a Glance

To avoid eating at fast food or convenience stores as much as possible, try these ideas:

* **Plan ahead and stash your own healthy "fast foods"** in the car, at work, and other places where you might be tempted to grab a quick meal. If you have to dash out for something quick, the best fast food is the kind you grab from your local grocer: whole fruits, salads made at the bar (dressed in vinegar and spices), and, depending on the establishment, some of the options at the hot bar.

* **When you have no choice but to grab a quick meal on the go, choose fast vegetables over fast meat.** A vegetable-stuffed submarine sandwich that is devoid of lunch meat can often be found even at most rest stops. Just make sure to hold the cheese and pair it with water or iced tea rather than a soft drink. Other restaurants offer salads, baked potatoes, grilled portobello sandwiches, fruit cups, and other choices.

* **Ask a lot of questions,** especially when ordering seemingly healthy-sounding wraps and sandwiches. The creamy glop they use as a sauce can sometimes contain more calories and fat than most people realize.

* **Look for a restaurant that makes fruit smoothies from real fruits and vegetables** and not from a mix. Smoothie mixes contain mostly sugar and very little fruit. Fresh juice bars are popping up in many places, and fresh vegetable-based choices can be very filling and nutritious.

Power Rx: If You Eat Meat, Avoid Hormones and Antibiotics

I gave up meat many years ago, and I'd love if everyone else did the same. That said, I know the idea of forgoing animal products sounds like a steep change for many. A great first step: Make sure the meat you do eat is as naked as possible. By naked, I mean clean—meat that contains no antibiotics, hormones, sodium, artificial colors, nitrites, pesticides, or hidden additives. If you buy meat at the supermarket, you can look for labels like "hormone and antibiotic free." One better: buy meat straight from the farmer. That way you can ask questions about how the animal was raised and butchered.

In addition to being free of hormones and antibiotics, you also want to buy meat that comes from animals that dined on grass or other natural food sources, not meat that comes from animals that consumed grain from a feedlot. That's because meat from grass-fed animals has more healthy omega-3 fatty acids.

But I understand that it can sometimes be tough to find clean meat and certainly more expensive to buy. So if you really can't go 100 percent for clean meat, at the very least make a goal of banning processed meat from your dinner plate. By processed, I'm talking about meat that has been preserved by smoking, curing, salting, or chemical preservatives. In other words: ham, bacon, sausages, hot dogs, and luncheon meats.

I don't care if that dog is made from chicken instead of beef or if that sausage is turkey. I don't care if the package of bacon says it's "nitrite free." In three words: Don't eat it.

Processed meats are the most deadly type of meat you could possibly ingest. When British researchers studied the food habits and health outcomes of 448,568 men and women, they found that people who ate the most processed meat (from lunch meat, hot dogs, bacon, and other sources) were more likely to die over the course of the study than people who consumed less. They were also more likely to have heart disease and cancer. The researchers estimated that three percent of all deaths could have been prevented had those people held their processed meat consumption to less than 20 grams a day.[58] That's the amount in half a slice of bacon!

Harvard researchers have also found that every 1.8 ounces of processed meats you eat raises your risk of heart disease by a whopping 42 percent. Think about that the next time you have a hankering for one of those hot dogs that seem to be rotating on permanent display in gas station delis.[59]

Why are processed meats so deadly? Sodium (processed meats contain four times more blood-pressure-raising sodium than unprocessed meat) and nitrite preservatives. Unlike the nitrates that come from plants, nitrites have been shown to promote hardening of the arteries and to hinder blood sugar control.

Rx at a Glance

If you choose to eat meat, insist on the best quality of fish and meat (wild-caught, grass-fed and free of hormones, GMOs, and antibiotics). Look for beef labeled "no hormones, no antibiotics, grass-fed." Avoid cuts labeled "vegetarian diet," as these cows often dine on grain as well as grass. It can be hard to find fish not contaminated with mercury and pesticides like DDT, but wild-caught fish from reputable suppliers are available. While it's true that higher-quality meat costs less per pound, I suggest that you eat less meat per meal so you aren't spending more overall.

Of course, there will be some times when lower quality meat might seem like your only option. Perhaps you're traveling. Perhaps your mother-in-law serves her world famous chicken cordon bleu while you're visiting. Whatever the reasons, protect your heart with this advice:

* **Always consume vegetables or fruit with any type of meat,** and especially with conventionally raised meat. The healing plant chemicals naturally present in fruits and vegetables might buffer some of the harmful effects of meat. Make the vegetables and fruits the biggest portion of your dinner plate, and meat the garnish.

* **Use spices at every meal,** especially if you'll be eating meat. Spices have natural anti-inflammatory actions, and can help offset any inflammatory foods in your meat. Turmeric root especially, and its component curcumin, act to suppress inflammation and promote health. Curry powder contains a combination of healing spices, including turmeric, hot red pepper, and cumin. If you are traveling, pack a small container of curry powder and sprinkle it on your restaurant meals.

* **Keep your serving of meat as small as possible,** using it more as an accent than the main course. Fill in around it with plant-based side dishes.

* **If you're grilling meat, marinate it first** to avoid AGE byproducts. These are formed when meat is cooked under high, dry heat, and they AGE every cell in your body.

Power Rx: If You Eat Meat, Consume It Only after Dark

As I just told you, processed meats rank as the worst animal products you can consume. Unfortunately, that doesn't mean that everything else from the meat kingdom is good for your heart.

Because of the endotoxin and AGEs that lurk in all forms of meat—even skinless, organic chicken breast—animal products are a food group you'll want to minimize.

Many people think of chicken as a health food, but much of the chicken available at your grocery store is actually mass produced in awful surroundings and requires cleansing in chlorine and arsenic, and often irradiation, to lower the risk of *E. coli* infections. This is so far removed from the farm-fresh approach of 50 to 100 years ago that it may sicken you spiritually and physically as it does me. And, as with all animal products, chicken contains AGEs, harmful substances that only proliferate when you cook it.

It's the same with dairy. Dairy foods are the number one source of heart vessel–clogging saturated fat in the diet. Conventionally produced milk also contains many different contaminants, including pesticides, growth hormones, and antibiotics.

But you're probably wondering: What about my bones? Don't I need to drink milk in order to have strong bones? Not necessarily. The Nurses' Health Study found that women who consumed 2.5 or more servings of dairy a day had the same risk of bone fractures as women who consumed fewer servings.[60]

And when Australian researchers compared the bone densities of 105 vegan Buddhist nuns to 105 non-vegetarians, they found no difference between the two groups. The nuns had bones that were just as strong as the milk drinkers'.[61]

And now let's talk about eggs. The yolk of just one egg has 185 milligrams of cholesterol, more than half of the maximum amount the American Heart Association recommends any of us consume in an entire day. Eggs are also a rich source of lecithin, which gut bacteria convert to TMAO (trimethylamine N-oxide), a possible harmful chemical. In one study, people with the highest levels of TMAO in their blood had 2.5 times the risk of suffering a heart attack. And a Canadian study of more than a thousand people found that the regular consumption of egg yolks is almost as damaging to the arteries as smoking. People who ate three or more yolks a week had more heart plaque than people who only had two or fewer yolks a week. Eggs are particularly dangerous for people who have diabetes, with one daily egg increasing the risk of also developing heart disease two- to fivefold, found the study.[62, 63]

Most of my patients aren't quite willing to go vegan cold turkey (pun intended). Despite the mounting evidence of meat's harmful attributes, many people still want to have at least some meat in their lives. If you feel the same, I understand that right now you are not ready to fully leap into the green, healthy life that is best for you. Healthy eating is a journey and you may be on your way to better and healthier choices. That's why I suggest you follow food journalist Mark Bittman's rule from his latest book *Eat Vegan Before 6:00* or, put another way, "Eat Animals after Dark." By following this rule, you limit your consumption of animal products to one meal a day, and that is for all eggs, dairy, and meat of any kind. If you are like most people, this rule will automatically slash your animal product consumption by roughly two-thirds.

Rx at a Glance

When eating any animal after dark, use these pointers:

* **Make breakfast, lunch, and snacks 100 percent plant based.**

* **Consume meat only at dinner,** holding your serving size to no more than 4 ounces: roughly the size of a pack of playing cards. If you stick to this amount once a day, you'll be able to avoid many of the health problems associated with Western-style rampant meat eating. One easy way to automatically consume the right-sized meat portion: Divide your dinner plate into fourths. Dedicate one-half of the plate to vegetables and fruits, with the emphasis on brightly colored fresh produce. Reserve one-quarter for grains. The last

quarter of the plate, only 25 percent, can be left open for meat.

* **Choose only one animal product at a time.** That means it's either meat or eggs or milk. It's not all three. Both eggs and dairy contain heart-harming ingredients, so it's just as important to minimize them as it is other types of meat.

Does this sound like too big of a change? Then slowly transition into it rather than doing it all at once. Swap one weekly meat-based meal for a non-meat-based one. Then do another. And another. Many of my patients say breakfast is the easiest meal to make over, so you might want to start there. Instead of an omelet filled with sausage, opt for one that contains only vegetables. Eventually swap out the omelet for a plant-based breakfast: oatmeal (one of the few packaged foods that earn an endorsement from the American Heart Association), an apple or banana smeared with natural peanut butter (bonus points if you grind it yourself or buy a brand in a glass jar), or a bowl of fruit sprinkled with cinnamon, coupled with fresh veggie juice.

Once you've made over breakfast, move on to lunch by gravitating toward huge salads, veggie wraps, bean soups, and other plant-based fare.

Then, for extra credit, go meatless some nights of the week as well, substituting any of the following healthy protein choices in for meat: beans, nuts, seeds, tempeh, seitan, and tofu. I am reticent to recommend fish to my patients because of the health risks now present in most sources of seafood. Frankly, the oceans are now dirty places that have been contaminated from years of us humans dumping pesticides and chemicals in our lakes, rivers, and streams. However, fish are a concentrated source of anti-inflammatory omega-3 essential fatty acids like DHA and EPA, so they can be a heart-healthy alternative to red meat and poultry. Follow the next prescription to maximize the benefits and minimize the risks of eating fish.

Power Rx: Swap SMASH Fish in for Meat

Certain types of fish account for your richest sources of omega-3 fatty acids, a heart-healthy essential fatty acid (EFA). Omega-3 fatty acids are important because they are known to reduce inflammation, heart rhythm disturbances, triglyceride levels, and high blood pressure. Diets rich in this EFA might also prevent plaque from building up in your arteries.

The fish that are richest in omega-3 fatty acids tend to swim in very cold waters, such as salmon, anchovies, and herring. If you can think of the word SMASH, then these fish are easy to remember: Sardines, Mackerel, Anchovies, Salmon, Herring. Be very careful to avoid farm-raised fish, as their growing conditions are horrible. Also, as GMO-raised fish enter the market, steer clear!

When getting your omega-3 fatty acids, however, you want to try to avoid accidentally consuming a heavy metal called mercury. Mercury has pervaded the environment mostly due to coal-burning power plants. It has seeped into our oceans, where it accumulates in the bodies of fish. The smallest of fish tend to have the lowest amounts. Mercury becomes more concentrated as you move up the fish food chain, with big fish having the most.

It is possible to eat enough fish, particularly sushi, to achieve high blood levels of mercury and become acutely ill. There is no healthy function for mercury in the body. Unfortunately, mercury inactivates some of the body's most important natural antioxidants, leaving the arteries exposed to oxygen damage. Mercury may also poison important enzymes in our mitochondria, the powerhouses of our cells, reducing energy production and directly damaging the lining of arteries by reducing an important healthy chemical called nitric oxide. Excess mercury is related to high blood pressure, heart attacks, stroke, and hardening of arteries.

Rx at a Glance

If you are eating fish, reduce your consumption to twice a week, particularly of large fish like sharks that have a high concentration of mercury. To do so:

* **Avoid sushi tuna,** which tends to be much higher in mercury than canned tuna.
* **Avoid large fish** like swordfish, shark, king mackerel, and tilefish.
* **Choose smaller fish.** Varieties that tend to be low in mercury include shrimp, canned light tuna, salmon, pollock, and catfish.

Power Rx: Temporarily Take a Break from Dairy and Wheat

Occasionally patients will come to me who are seemingly doing everything right. They are exercising, eating plenty of vegetables, and meditating so regularly that they are as calm as a lake on a wind-free day.

Still, when I test their blood for markers of inflammation, the labs will come back high.

And that's when I start suspecting a food allergy or intolerance. Undiagnosed food allergies and intolerances are one of the hidden causes of inflammation, and allergies to dairy and wheat top the list. Eggs, nuts, shellfish, fish, corn, and soy round out the list of other common food allergens that could be a source of inflammation and poor health and also might be worth avoiding for at least a while.

Before coming to see me, it never occurred to many of my patients that their frequent stomachaches and fatigue were the result of an allergy or intolerance.

Our bodies react the same way to allergens as they do to

poisons and other irritants. As a result, inflammation increases whenever we eat these foods.

First, let's take a close look at wheat. It is important to understand that wheat has changed in the last century and has become a more complex structure. The original form of wheat, einkorn wheat, had a simple genetic makeup of only 14 chromosomes (we humans have 46, by the way). Humans evolved on this type of wheat, and, for thousands of years, it's what we cultivated.

Modern-day wheat, however, called triticum wheat, is the result of purposeful breeding experiments to increase the yield of wheat crops. Today's triticum wheat may have as many as 42 chromosomes and grows shorter and sturdier for greater yield.

In our bodies, the gluten protein in this newer triticum wheat may irritate our digestive tracts. A few studies have shown that gluten protein directly stimulates the release of zonulin in the gut. Zonulin is a protein that regulates the permeability of the intestines.

Elegant research done by my colleague Alessio Fasano, MD, at Harvard Medical School, shows that these tight junctions can be loosened in some sensitive people by the chronic ingestion of gluten and dairy.[64] Once the tight junctions are no longer tight, bowel contents can leak into the bloodstream. This isn't a good thing because your bloodstream is not equipped to handle partially digested food, toxins, and the other contents of your GI tract. When small amounts seep into the bloodstream, the immune system goes on high alert and you experience chronic inflammation. This is called a leaky gut and may be the most common cause of chronic illnesses.

Imagine your bowl of breakfast cereal causing your colon to leak like a vegetable strainer!

If you are intolerant, it's the same story with dairy and other possible trigger foods. These allergies and intolerances often have been with patients for years, but the symptoms are mild and come and go.

Rx at a Glance

Does everyone need to give up dairy and wheat? For reasons I've already mentioned (see page 114), I heartily recommend that everyone give up dairy, but it's especially important for people who are lactose intolerant. As for wheat, though, it depends. Many studies and organizations have linked whole grains with better heart health. So if you're not sensitive to wheat, you don't need to give it up. Here's an easy way to find out if you're intolerant to dairy or wheat:

* **Take a vacation from either dairy or wheat, abstaining for about three to four weeks.** During that time use non-dairy alternatives like coconut milk or gluten-free foods, depending on which food group you gave up.

* **After four weeks, note how you feel.** Many of my patients tell me that after taking a dairy and/or wheat vacation they feel better than they have in years. That's a good sign that you have an intolerance to one or both of these foods.

If you noticed no improvement, you're probably fine. Work that food back in, and then eliminate the other one and see how you feel.

Power Rx: Go Vegan

Years ago when I was a resident physician, I read John Robbins's *Diet for a New America,* and it forever changed what I eat. His description of the deplorable conditions that cattle, pigs, and chickens must endure turned my stomach and I no longer could bring myself to eat foods from industries that had resulted in such intense suffering.

Over the years, I've learned that what I originally started doing for moral and spiritual reasons was also improving my health. That's why I now recommend a vegan diet (whole food, plant based) to all my patients, and it's why I'm asking you to adopt one, too. When you follow a healthy whole food vegan diet, you naturally consume a heart-healthy bounty of fiber, healing plant chemicals, minerals, vitamins, and antioxidants, all of which work together to drop cholesterol, cool inflammation, and improve the health of every cell in your body. And, no, while Skittles for three meals a day might technically be vegan, that is not the whole food, plant-based diet I am talking about.

At the same time, you won't be eating the saturated fat, cholesterol, antibiotics, hormones, and other ingredients that cause animal products to raise inflammation throughout the body.

The world's longest-lived people—those who live in the "Blue Zones" of Okinawa, Japan; Ikaria, Greece; Nicoya, Costa Rica; Sardinia, Italy; and Loma Linda, California—all have something in common. The cornerstone of their diets is plants: beans, sweet potatoes, vegetables, fruit, and whole grains. And when scientists in Europe examined 13 years' worth of dietary records from hundreds of thousands of people, they found that the people who consumed the most fruits and vegetables (an average of a pound or more a day) had a 15 percent lower risk of dying than people who ate the fewest (less than a half pound a day.)[65] Those who benefited the most from this produce-rich diet? People who were obese, regular drinkers, and smokers.

Rx at a Glance

A vegan diet isn't for everyone, of course, but I couldn't end this chapter without suggesting it. If you are very motivated to improve your heart health—as former president Clinton was after his bypass surgery—then you'll probably find a vegan diet easy to adopt. If you are not as motivated, go slowly, taking small steps.

* **Buy vegan cookbooks,** subscribe to magazines (such as *Vegetarian Times*), and read vegan websites for cooking and meal-planning ideas.

* **Think of the foods you generally eat in a day and brainstorm creative ways to swap in plant-based foods** for meat-based ones. Maybe have peanut butter on your toast instead of butter, for instance. Or swap in marinara sauce for a meat-based one. Instead of a ham and cheese sandwich, you might opt for hummus and vegetables or avocado and eggplant.

* **Special order.** Many restaurants, I've found, are delighted to create a special vegan dish if you ask ahead, and vegan options are becoming more and more commonplace on menus.

* **Experiment.** You can blend tofu with various spices to create a cheese-like texture. It's the same with nutritional yeast.

YOUR FINAL NUTRITION RX

When I advise my patients, I take out my prescription pad and I write down rules to follow. I'm not sitting next to you inside your house, so I can't do the same for you.

But you can do it for yourself. Get a small piece of paper. On it write one prescription from this chapter that you plan to incorporate into your life. Maybe you plan to ditch soda (great one!) or maybe you're opting to eat animals after dark.

Whatever it is, write it down and put it on the fridge. That way you'll see it whenever you are in the kitchen and you are thinking about or preparing food.

Once you have that one change under control, try another one and another one. Don't fall into the trap of making perfect the enemy of good. Any small change moves your heart health in the right direction. So think about your current diet, the foods you love, and your lifestyle. What's a realistic change that you can make easily? Start with that. For instance, let's say you are very busy, and that, until you read this chapter, you practically lived

Ask the Holistic Heart Doc:
Is it really possible to find healthy vegan meals at a restaurant?

Yes, indeed, it is. Some types of restaurants are more likely to serve healthy vegan fare: Thai, Cal-Mex, Japanese, and Middle Eastern. And many chains now offer at least one vegan option, ranging from a veggie burger to a baked potato paired with a salad to tomato pie.

If there's nothing explicitly vegan on the menu, you still have options. You can veganize an existing dish—for instance, by ordering a grilled chicken salad without the chicken or a veggie pizza without the cheese. Or you can combine a number of small plates and/or side dishes, such as broccoli, a side of baked beans, and a baked potato. Just tell the wait staff that you are on President Bill Clinton's diet and ask for the same dish that they would prepare for him! It works for me.

This is what else I like to do. If I am dining out for a business meeting, I will always call ahead and ask to speak to the chef. I inform the chef of my desire for a plant-based, whole food, elegant meal that is low in fat. The results are amazing. Generally everyone at the table wants to know how I got the special plate of tasty morsels, and I am asked to share samples liberally.

Even at steak houses I've been served grilled portobello mushrooms, sautéed vegetables, bean dishes, and cheese-free risottos on a routine basis. On shorter notice, alerting a waiter of my desire to order without cheese, to use lemon juice or balsamic vinegar as a dressing, to substitute a side salad for fries, or to eat only vegetable side dishes is second nature and usually received politely. I do not intend it, but the steak and chicken eaters usually feel rather guilty and envious when they see my healthy plate!

Yes, you can order a pizza without cheese anywhere and just load it up with vegetables and marinara sauce (rich in lycopene, which is good for arteries and the prostate). When I ask for unsweetened items such as iced tea, this can usually be accommodated. When not available, something like low-salt V8 juice (if available, or if I packed it) will be my fare.

on fast food and diet soda. Perhaps your first step is going online so you can research the menus of various fast food restaurants. Instead of the double cheeseburger, perhaps you opt for a garden burger. Instead of the meatball sub, you have the veggie one. Or perhaps instead of a side of fries, you opt for the baby carrots.

Similarly, if you've been eating meat every day, three times a day, your first step might simply be research. Where can you buy naked meat in your area? Do any local farmers sell grass-fed, hormone- and antibiotic-free meat at a farmer's market? Do any of your local grocery stores stock it? How much does it cost? Make it your goal for at least half of the meat you consume to be free from unnecessary toxins. And go for at least one meat-free meal a day.

From there, you might reduce your meat consumption by adding chopped veggies, brown rice, pureed beans, and other foods to meatloaf, casseroles, and other meat-based dishes.

Over time, you might declare one day a week "meat free." Then another. Perhaps you subscribe to *Vegetarian Times* or another magazine for ideas on meat-free dinners.

The point is this: If you overwhelm yourself with too many changes, you may very well end up making no changes at all. So, no matter how seemingly minor, start with one small change, congratulate yourself on your effort, and make more changes from there.

Pick the changes that make the most sense for you and your lifestyle. I think you'll be pleasantly surprised to find that, once you start incorporating various prescriptions into your eating life, your health will improve dramatically. Soon you'll be feeling so good that you'll want to incorporate many more.

Chapter 7

Your Food Prep Rx

In the last chapter you learned *what* to eat—as well as what not to eat. Just remember a high P/A (more plants to fewer animals) ratio and you will have the most important lesson mastered.

In this chapter, you'll gain some important insights into *how* to eat. This chapter will help you put everything you just learned in Chapter 6 into practice. What you'll find in the following pages are prescriptions that are not taught in medical school. Most are based on cutting-edge science, and they are so new that you probably will not have heard about them from your health care provider, from the Internet, from other health books, or even from that friend who always seems to be in the know.

You might wonder: Why do you continually eat foods that you know are just not good for you? For instance, perhaps you've tried to change your diet many times before. You might have come away from those experiences thinking that you just don't have the motivation or inclination to change your diet. This just isn't true. In reality, you may have failed only because you didn't have the right appliances, advice, and cooking skills to make healthy eating convenient. Skill power helps willpower.

I'll let you in on a secret: You're not alone! Most people are too busy to cook daily meals that require an hour or more of preparation. Many more fall victim to temptation. They tell themselves that they will only snack on veggies and hummus and then end up eating fried snack chips instead.

Still, just as many very busy people—people who happen to love a good dessert or chip as much as the next one—still manage to consume an amazingly healthy diet. How do they do it? They use a handful of important strategies that allow them to reduce temptation for junk and also to make healthy eating more convenient. You'll find those strategies in this chapter.

You'll also find some amazing prescriptions that will help your body make the most of every important nutrient. *What you choose to eat is only half of the nutrition equation. How you shop for it, store it, cook it, and consume it matters just as much.*

Power Rx: Do a Clean Sweep of Your Kitchen

I was a big fan of the TV series *Clean Sweep* that used to air on TLC. On the show, an organizer, designer, and carpenter would clean out two rooms of someone's house, often tossing or donating most of the contents to charity.

I liked the show so much that I began wondering what would happen if everyone did a clean sweep of just one room of their homes: the kitchen. I soon began suggesting my patients do just that. I was amazed by how many of them took me up on it, and even more amazed when they reported back, telling me, "You will not believe all the stuff I got rid of!" When I asked them to search for boxed foods that had partially hydrogenated vegetable oils (trans fats), artificial sweeteners, high fructose corn syrup, chemicals they couldn't pronounce, and cans lined with bisphenol-A, they would come back to the office in shock because half of their pantry items were toxic to their health.

When you make a clean sweep of your kitchen, you accomplish

a lot more than creating a more organized eating environment. You also toss all the tempting foods that are bad for your heart, automatically increasing your chances of eating wholesome foods like fruits and vegetables.

Rx at a Glance

Take a tour of your pantry, refrigerator, and freezer. Pull out various food items and check out their labels. Toss or donate any item that contains:

* **Partially hydrogenated vegetable oils.**
* **High fructose corn syrup (HFCS).**
* **Sugar by any of its aliases:** dextrin, dextrose, glucose, honey, maltodextrin, malt syrup, maltose, saccharose, sorghum, sucrose, and any ingredient that includes the word "syrup."
* **Long lists of ingredients that you cannot pronounce** and that sound like a chemistry exam.
* **Items with health claims like "low-fat,"** which usually are super high in processed sugar and additives, creating inflammation.
* **Items in cans not marked "BPA-free."**
* **Anything bathed in four kinds of cheese.**

That's just for starters. Of course, there will probably be some foods that you are tempted to toss, but that one or more family members declare essential to taste bud survival. If that's the case, then strike a compromise. Store the artery-clogging food in an opaque container where it's not easy to find or see. Out of sight really can be out of mind. If you don't see the food every time you open a cabinet, you'll be less likely to eat it.

Molly's Journey to a Lasting Heart

When I walked into the exam room to talk to Molly about her high blood pressure and cholesterol, I could tell something was different. In the past, whenever she talked about her struggles with her voracious sweet tooth, she would avert her eyes, looking down in her lap. She'd admitted to keeping small candy bars in her car, desk, purse, and even her gym locker. Some days guilt won and she resisted them, but many days she would eat four or five. She then described how on those days she might add in a can of soda, a bag of chips, a deep dish pizza loaded with cheese, and a nighttime dessert. She felt out of control and her weight and blood pressure had not responded well for the last few years. With small children at home and a busy real estate job, she had little time to focus on her health.

On this visit, however, she looked me right in the eyes. I noticed a different hairstyle, brighter clothes, and some colorful jewelry. Before I could ask how she had been doing, she blurted out, "Doc, I finally got it—all you have been telling me on prior visits. When you pulled out your Rx pad last visit and wrote down a smoothie recipe and the three Killer Bs to purchase, I made a decision to listen."

Indeed I often take out my Rx pad and, rather than write a new medicine, I list a video to watch, a website or book to read, a supplement to buy, or a kitchen accessory to purchase. For Molly I had prescribed *Fat, Sick and Nearly Dead,* a video about the story of Joe Cross and how he transformed his life by juicing vegetables. I had referred her to his website of the same name and asked her to begin each day with a plant-packed juice or smoothie.

But you're probably wondering the most about the Killer Bs. If you're a wine lover, you may have heard the term used to refer to Italy's finest wines: Barolo, Babaresco, and Brunello. I have adopted the term to refer to three appliances that help you create healthier beverages:

- The Bullet (and other similar brands): Really called the NutriBullet, this small blender has very powerful blades and is often advertised on TV. It costs around $100, and makes cleanup super easy.

- The Breville (and other similar brands): This is a centrifugal juicer.
- The Blendtec (and other similar brands): This is a large, high-powered blender.

From my Rx pad Molly had researched and ordered a NutriBullet, and tried many of the recipes for homemade smoothies, juices, and dips that came with the device. She told me they were simple for her and cleanup was a breeze. "I haven't had a bowl of breakfast cereal since the Bullet arrived," she said. Instead, she'd had a blended bowl of salad for breakfast, masked as a tasty green-berry smoothie.

The Breville was a bigger decision. At first she did not want to spend the $250 or so, so she went to a local big box store and bought a lower-cost brand. She committed to juicing organic vegetables, fruits, and spices twice a week. Her children were intrigued and offered to help. They became a juicing team and soon they were using it four times a week. Sometimes she made a fruit juice like pure watermelon or orange, but her favorite was one with cucumber, celery, apples, kale, greens, lemon, and ginger. After four months her husband surprised her with the more powerful Breville, and she was sold.

Finally she decided to replace her 22-year-old blender with a more powerful modern model. She looked at the Blendtec and the Vitamix, both the top of the line. Both had powerful motors and could make soups and family dishes. She decided on the Vitamix and has become adept at making cold and hot soups, sauces, fruit sorbet, and other treats.

She told me that she made it a habit to grocery shop for fresh produce twice a week, and, as a result, her refrigerator had been transformed from a meat morgue to a vegetable stand. She made a big pot of brown rice and soup twice a week and, when in a pinch, now always had some of those prepared foods to pack for the office or to eat on the run. And the best news? She had lost 14 pounds, her blood pressure was normal, and her cholesterol had fallen 30 mg/dl.

Power Rx: Shop Along the Edges of the Grocery Store

Once you've emptied out your kitchen cabinets, it's time to shop for heart-healthy foods to stock instead.

As it turns out, how you shop at the grocery store is just as important as what you shop for. If you are like most people and aimlessly wander down every single aisle, it's likely you'll toss into your cart many of the very foods you just tossed from your kitchen. This is especially true if you shop on an empty stomach, by the way.

To reduce the call of tempting processed foods, my recommendation here is a simple one: Shop along the edges of the grocery store as much as possible. That's where you will find whole foods: vegetables and fruit. These foods rarely come encased in plastic (see Chapter 10), and usually don't have nutritional labels that list word after unfamiliar word. On the other hand, it's the middle of the store where you'll find the tempting processed foods that have been encased in plastic bags that have then been stuffed into cardboard boxes. Some of these foods are so far from the tree that it's hard to guess the original plant that was used to make them.

Rx at a Glance

Of course, there are some foods in the middle that you'll feel you have to have, whether it's for convenience or for health. Use this advice when venturing into the middle:

* **Never shop while hungry.** It's rare for a hungry person to walk into the middle aisles of the grocery store and manage to emerge with a heart-healthy option.

* **Don't get duped by marketing.** Many products claim to be "whole grain," but that doesn't make them healthy. If it sounds too good to be true—as it is in the case of "whole grain corn chips"—it probably is.

* **Whenever possible, look for products and packaging labeled "BPA-free."** If a product isn't labeled, check out the code on the plastic container. Bottles marked with recycle code 7 are the most likely to contain BPA and should be avoided. Codes 3 and 6 can contain other toxins and should be avoided as well. Codes 1, 2, 4, and 5 are less likely to be dangerous.

* **Always read the list of ingredients, even if a product claims to be "trans-fat free."** If a product lists partially hydrogenated vegetable oil, skip it. The same is true if you see the following words: high fructose corn syrup, MSG (monosodium glutamate), and any chemical preservatives that you can't pronounce. Look for alternative brands that either don't contain those ingredients at all or, at the very least, list them much farther down the list of ingredients. Single- or minimal-ingredient foods are the best choice.

* **Look for a non-GMO label on products with corn, soy, and canola.**

* **If possible, rather than bring your cart from aisle to aisle as you look for those foods, keep it safely stationed in the major, perimeter cart freeway.** Then walk to the item you need from the middle of the store, grab it, and walk back to the cart. Without your cart there on the ready, you'll be less tempted to grab other not-so-wholesome foods that happen to be stocked in the same aisle.

* **Hold your middle-aisle foraging to wholesome foods** like BPA-free canned beans, canned chopped tomatoes, frozen fruit, oatmeal, spices, raw nuts and seeds, and bagged or boxed grains like quinoa, amaranth, flax, chia seed, and wild rice.

Power Rx: Break the Record for the Person Who Eats the Slowest

In the previous chapter, I told you how certain types of vegetables—especially salad greens like arugula and spinach—contain a substance that converts to nitric oxide in the body, helping to dilate blood vessels and lower blood pressure.

It's important that, whenever you eat, you savor your food slowly, making sure to thoroughly chew every bite. Chewing slowly and completely allows the beginning of the breakdown of nutrients to enhance the absorption of vitamins, minerals, and other nutrients. It allows the nitrates in your salad to interact with the enzymes and bacteria in your mouth, converting nitrates into nitrites.

Chewing slowly also provides some other benefits. For one, you'll eat less automatically. As I've already mentioned, excess body weight raises your risk for heart disease. Eating slowly can help you to slim down, somewhat effortlessly. There's a 20-minute lag between the stomach filling with food and the brain getting the "I'm full" message. If you eat hurriedly, you'll consume many hundreds of unneeded calories. If you eat slowly, your brain will register fullness many bites of food sooner.

Here's another important reason to slow down: pleasure. I don't know about you, but I used to find myself rushing through a meal. The meal would end and I would think, "Who came in here and ate my lunch? I don't remember eating any of that." Now when I take time to savor my food, I find I enjoy the entire eating experience so much more. As a result, I feel satisfied after eating much less.

Rx at a Glance

Use these tips to train yourself to eat more slowly:

* **Get rid of the distractions.** It's difficult to slow down when your mind is occupied elsewhere. Turn off the TV and ditch the smartphone. And sit down.

* **Pause before eating.** Perhaps you say grace or maybe you sit quietly, thinking about how fortunate you are to have access to three meals a day. Or maybe you just take a few, slow breaths.

* **At the very least, make a conscious effort to savor the first three bites,** thoroughly chewing each one. Then make it your goal to do the same with the last three.

* **Eat with your non-dominant hand or try chopsticks.** Both tactics will naturally slow you down.

* **Place your flatware down between bites.**

Power Rx: Tune In to the Pleasure of Eating

Mindfulness is a stress reduction practice that has been used successfully in people with heart disease. Tuning in to the present moment helps to take you out of the past (where guilt, regret, and anger reside) and the future (the birthplace of anxiety). As you'll learn in coming chapters, the more you can reduce stress, anger, and anxiety, the healthier your heart. Being mindful and grateful for what you are eating and how you eat it is a core tenet of many religions and a great health practice you can start right now.

The more mindful you are of the smell, taste, sight, and texture of your food, the more likely it is that you will enjoy it and the less likely it is that you will overeat.

Rx at a Glance

Mindfulness is a great way to train yourself to enjoy all of the healthy foods that you are now eating. Here are some ways to do it:

* **Before taking the first bite, visually take in what your meal looks like on your plate.** Notice how it smells, too. And take a moment to feel grateful that you have such delicious food to eat. How wonderful!

* **Think about all of the ways that meal will help you live longer.** As you chew and swallow, imagine the nutrients traveling into your cells, where they heal inflammation and reverse heart disease.

* **Chew slowly and savor the unique texture of your food.**

Power Rx: Do Your Own Food Prep

One of the best ways to avoid many of the pitfalls I warned you about in Chapter 6 is to cook your own food. Yet so few people do. As a result, many of us have become enslaved by the convenience food industry, feeling at the mercy of the very unhealthy foods marketed to us at the grocery store and fast food establishments.

And cooking your own food doesn't require a degree in culinary science. Even if you don't know the difference between a butcher's knife and a paring knife, you can get the hang of preparing your own meals. Stock up on cookbooks, cooking magazines, and cooking websites. These will inspire you to act. Then, surround yourself with friends who cook. Again, they'll motivate you to spend more time in your kitchen. Finally, prepare. The hardest part of cooking isn't figuring out what to put in the frying pan. No, it's thinking ahead and making sure you actually have something on hand to cook up for breakfast, lunch, or dinner.

Rx at a Glance

Here's what I do to make sure I don't need to stop off for fast food or resort to buying foods made in plants:

* **Wake up 15 minutes earlier** to cook some steel-cut oats with walnuts, blend up a berry green smoothie with rice milk, or eat some fruit.

* **Prepare lunches the night before,** making stews, soups, and rice dishes, for example, that can last for two to three days or more. Make this a routine.

* **Have healthy snacks of nuts, seeds and fresh fruit in your office, car, or briefcase** so you can fight the urge to reach for the muffin or doughnut sitting in the break room.

* **Spend as much time planning your food as you do planning a golf trip or an outing with children.**

* **When you go on road trips, bring a cooler full of food along.** That way your stomach won't be held captive by the paltry options available at most rest stops.

* **Before traveling anywhere, consult HappyCow.net** to find restaurants in the area that serve up healthy fare.

* **When eating out, order three vegetable side dishes** rather than one meal. I, for instance, have been known to order corn, spinach, and a salad. It's not

glamorous, but it keeps my heart healthy. I've also had awesome black-eyed peas and greens in the South that didn't have a drop of animal protein or fat.

Power Rx: Avoid Heart AGErs with Smart Cooking Techniques

You can quickly turn any type of meat into a heart ager if you cook it under dry, high heat, such as in the microwave or on the grill. You can, on the other hand, render your meat more heart healthy simply by cooking with moisture, such as by braising or steaming. It really does make a difference, and here's why.

All meats—no matter what kind of animal they come from—are natural sources of substances called advanced glycation end products (AGEs), also known as glycotoxins, in the body. AGEs are some of the chemicals most dangerous to the human body, and they do exactly what their name implies. They age you, causing stiff muscles, wrinkles, and inflammation. AGEs stiffen your blood vessels, raising blood pressure. They can also erode the blood vessel walls, leading to strokes. Our bodies have natural defense mechanisms in place to handle AGEs, but they work slowly. Over time, if too many AGEs come in, not enough go out. They build up, causing premature aging.

When researchers feed mice diets rich in AGEs, the rodents develop heart and kidney disease. When researchers restrict these substances, mice are less likely to develop heart disease and diabetes. Insulin sensitivity improves, and so does wound healing. The animals also live longer.[66]

No matter how many AGEs your food contains, you can send those levels sky high with the wrong cooking method. Dry heat accelerates the formation of new AGEs by 10 to 100 times. For example, grilled or broiled chicken and chicken nuggets have up to 10 times the amount of AGEs of boiled chicken. Even a fried egg has 50 times the AGE level of a boiled egg.

Rx at a Glance

Vegetarian diets are naturally very low in AGEs. However, if you eat only a small amount of meat—and you cook it in a heart-smart way—AGEs might not be a problem for you.

Use these tips to AGE more slowly over dinner:

* **Whenever possible, cook with moist heat instead of dry.** The presence of water helps to slow the formation of AGEs. Steam instead of sear, boil instead of microwave, braise instead of roast, and poach instead of grill.

* **If you're going to grill, marinate meat before and during cooking.** Moistened meats produce half the AGEs of dry meats. Lemon juice, vinegar, and dark beer make for particularly good marinade ingredients. Also, if you wrap foods in foil, you'll keep them moist during grilling, reducing some of the harmful AGEs.

* **Cook for shorter times at lower heat.** Avoid the high flames from extra lighter fluids and dripping fats.

* **Clean your grill.** Keeping the grill clean of old burnt residues or grilling on tinfoil may help avoid charring.

* **Have a vegetable quota.** Every night at dinner, I try to consume two to three servings of vegetables and fruits. The antioxidants and other healing chemicals in these foods help to counterbalance any AGEs I might have consumed earlier. I have them either raw, steamed, or lightly sautéed at low temperatures in vegetable broth.

* **Consider supplements.** The following supplements might block some of the ill effects of AGEs: benfotiamine (150 to 200 mg once a day), carnosine (250 to 500 mg once a day), and alpha-lipoic acid (300 to 600 mg once a day).

Power Rx: Drink Your Veggies

In the previous chapter, I suggested you consume a minimum of five servings of fruits and vegetables a day—and the more, the better, with health warriors exceeding 10 servings a day. (Feel free to push it to one or two pounds a day like the heroes on *The Biggest Loser* show.) Doing so requires a lot of slicing, dicing, and chewing. It's time-consuming. That's why I recommend you drink some of your veggies.

I began juicing on a regular basis after watching the food documentary *Fat, Sick and Nearly Dead*. This movie tells the story of an overweight Australian, Joe Cross, and his journey across America with a juicer. His health increased and his weight decreased dramatically by adding all the vitamins, minerals, antioxidants, and phytonutrients provided by vegetable juice.

It made me realize how a "mean green" juice can be such a convenient way to get several servings of vegetables. An eight-ounce glass of freshly prepared, green-based juice a day is an awesome way to increase your nutrition and have a healthy heart. Even if you can only manage this a few times a week, go for it. If it is fruit you want, eat it whole and get the fiber and avoid the store-bought sugary juices.

Rx at a Glance

To get more juiced vegetables into your life, use this advice:

* **Know your juicer.** Most juicers are called "centrifugal," and brands like Jack LaLanne and Breville have powerful motors that quickly shred a large pile of veggies and fruits to juice. They do heat up the juice a bit, and some experts say this heat might cause some loss of nutrition. There is another type called a macerating juicer, such as Omega, and they slowly grind the contents to juice, preserving more of the

nutrients. If you have ever seen wheatgrass squeezed into the emerald green juice that is so healing, you know of a macerating juicer. These juicers can take a long time to work their magic, so some people are frustrated by them. If you have more patience, they are a great option.

* **Add some wheatgrass to any juice you make.** One to two ounces of this chlorophyll-dense juice is the mainstay of many healing programs for inflammatory disorders. The best source of wheatgrass is freshly cut, either from grass you grow yourself or from a tray at a health food store. I tend to get mine from an enterprising couple who fought cancer with juicing and who have since started a wheatgrass greenhouse in my area. Check to see if there is a similar business in your area. They deliver freshly cut bags of the nutritious greens to our home. If you cannot find it fresh, there are sources that harvest the grass, juice it, freeze it, and ship it frozen to your home in bulk. Finally, you can buy powdered or tablet forms of wheatgrass that may be most practical when traveling.

* **Use roughly 60 percent veggies, 40 percent fruit when you start juicing.** As you gain experience and as your tastes allow, cut back on fruit even more until it is less than 20 percent. Vegetables are naturally low in sugar and calories. Fruit, on the other hand, is richer in both, so when you concentrate it into a juice, it can spike blood sugar. To sweeten up the juice, however, feel free to add a green apple or some berries.

  One exception to my advice about minimizing fruit: pomegranates. This fruit and its juice boost the level and function of the enzyme paraoxanase in the healthy HDL lipoprotein particle, helping shrink plaque in arteries. I add pomegranate juice or seeds to my morning smoothie every day.

* **Add healing spices to your juice.** They'll do more than liven up your drink. Turmeric, cumin, sage, ginger, garlic, basil, rosemary, sage, and hot peppers all have established medical benefits.

* **Drink your freshly made juice right away.** Fresh juice is highly perishable. Downing your juice right after it has come out of the juicer ensures you consume the most nutrients.

Dr. Kahn's Shot of Green Goodness

2	organic cucumbers
1	complete stalk of organic celery with the leaves on
1	lemon, whole
	Raw ginger, about 2 to 3 inches long
1	organic green apple
2 to 3	raw turmeric roots
1	handful of cilantro
1	handful of parsley
¼ to ½	pound fresh sprouts like broccoli, pea, or bean (when available)

This should fill about two Mason jars with green juice.

Power Rx: Chew Your Fruit (Avoid Fruit Juice)

I just suggested you drink fresh vegetable juice. Why not make fruit juices, too?

Vegetables are lower in sugar than fruits, so you don't have to worry about your blood sugar going crazy when you condense them into a drink.

But fruit is naturally richer in sugar. So when you blend it, you concentrate the sugar, creating a calorie-packed drink that has the ability to drive up your blood sugar. But when you eat fruit whole, it's not as concentrated. It has the toxin (sugar) and the antidote (fiber) packaged together. Exceptions like store-bought pomegranate juice, tart cherry juice, and perhaps low-sugar grape juice, which are loaded with polyphenols and anti-inflammatory chemicals, are great additions to smoothies.

More and more higher-quality, cold-pressed juices in glass or non–bisphenol-A bottles are showing up in stores—even at Starbucks and Costco. This trend is a major advance for a shot of nutrition on the run. Be careful to read the ingredients. Many of these are rich in fruit juice and very high in sugar and should be avoided if possible. On the other hand, brands like BluePrint, Drought, Suja, and Evolution Fresh have selections that are all or mainly vegetable. If you are purchasing bottled juices for your health, I recommend spending extra money to buy juices made from organic produce (and it's best if they're made mainly with green vegetables).

Rx at a Glance

When in doubt, use this rule of the nutritional thumb: Eat the fruit, juice (or eat) the vegetable. If a smoothie is your only option, follow this advice:

* **Ask a lot of questions.** Make sure the smoothie was made from real fruit rather than a fruit blend or mix.

* **Better yet, make your own.** Use dark berries (often called "brain berries" for their beneficial effect on memory) from the freezer, a scoop of "green" powders that contains vegetable grasses (such as chlorella or wheatgrass), and a protein source such as rice and pea protein powders, a dark leafy green such as kale or spinach, and some fresh-made juice or almond milk, to taste.

* **Avoid store-bought juice.** With a few key exceptions, most have been sitting around for up to a couple years, and they also contain many additives. If you are going to have fruit juice, make sure it's fresh squeezed from real fruit and loaded with the pulp.

Power Rx: Cook Once, Eat Five Times

Many of my patients are busy people. They work incredibly long days, and they come home to an active family life. When I ask them about what they eat, I learn that much of their food intake revolves around frozen dinners, pre-packaged convenience foods, fast foods, and eating out. They do very little true cooking.

"I can't cook healthy foods. I just don't have time," they tell me.

My prescription: a multi-use blender. It just might be the most important appliance you will ever buy for your health, and it's even more convenient and much healthier than your microwave! Make sure it's a high-quality blender such as a Blendtec or Vitamix brand.

Rx at a Glance

Your blender allows you to cook huge meals such as soups and stews only once or twice a week. No matter what you blend, it will last a few days in the fridge. And if you freeze some, it's like making your own frozen dinners. I love to toss the ingredients for cold soups such as gazpacho into my blender, but simple hot soups such as chili or minestrone are great, too. Try my Blender Delicious Tortilla Soup recipe on page 143; it's one of my favorites.

Your blender can also mix up large amounts of hummus and other healthy spreads to use on sandwiches or as a dip for vegetables. Use these tips:

* **Make batches of vegetable broth ahead of time.** Or, in a pinch, buy it in BPA-free cartons at the store. Use it as the base for any soup.

* **Add spices like curry powder or an Italian herb mix** to turn any quick soup into a creation that not only tastes like gourmet food but also offers powerful heart protection.

* **Always add green leafy vegetables to your broth, too.** If you have sprouts, they are also a great addition.

* **Use silken tofu to thicken soup,** giving it a creamy texture.

* **Add chunky ingredients such as beans at the end,** once you are done blending.

* **Couple your blender creation with other convenient grab-and-go fare** such as a leftover bean burger, a cooked potato or yam (both of which are easy to make ahead in large batches), or a large salad and perhaps a glass of red wine. Voila! Dinner is served. As always, if you do not have a blender yet or have not yet weaned yourself from the Standard American Diet (SAD for short and for sure), then remember the Golden Rule: Balance bad with good and add some fresh vegetables to your plate.

In addition to a blender, other appliances might help you consume heart-healthier meals. Leading the pack is a slow cooker. This wonderful invention allows you to toss in ingredients in the morning and come home to a delicious ready-to-eat meal. Another nice option: a huge casserole dish. There are hundreds of ways to cook healthy casseroles, and just one of them can last your family a few days, reducing your need to cook night after night.

Blender Delicious Tortilla Soup

3 cups (720 ml) vegetable broth
1 Roma tomato, halved, or about ½ cup chopped
1 carrot, halved, or about ½ cup chopped
1 rib celery, halved, or about ⅓ cup chopped
1 thin slice of onion, peeled, or approximately 1 tablespoon chopped
1 garlic clove, peeled
1 thin slice of yellow squash
1 thin slice of red bell pepper
1 thin slice of cabbage
1 mushroom

1 teaspoon taco seasoning
A dash of ground cumin
Salt and ground black pepper, to taste
½ cup (70 g) cooked chicken breast (optional)
½ fresh jalapeño
¼ cup olives, pitted
¼ cup (50 g) canned corn, unsalted
2 ounces (60 g) GMO-free tortilla chips

1. Place the broth, tomato, carrot, celery, onion, garlic, squash, bell pepper, cabbage, mushroom, taco seasoning, cumin, salt, and black pepper into your blender and secure the lid.

2. Select the lowest speed. Turn the machine on and slowly increase the speed to high. Blend for 5 to 6 minutes.

3. Reduce the speed to low and then tun the blender off. Remove the lid. Drop in the chicken (if using), jalapeño, olives, corn, and chips. On low speed, blend for 5 to 10 seconds and then serve.

Power Rx: Fast 11 Hours Every Night

Few people realize it, but they fast every single day. They don't feel deprived because they sleep through the entire experience. That's why we call our morning meal breakfast—it breaks the fast that started the night before, after the conclusion of dinner.

Breakfast is potentially the most important meal you can possibly consume, both for your metabolism and for your heart health. But here's something you may not know: It's just as important to eat a true break-fast. In other words, to fast for a period of time.

Researchers followed more than 26,000 male health professionals for 16 years, all the while tracking what they ate. At the conclusion of the study the men who skipped breakfast were 27 percent more likely to suffer a heart attack or death than those who ate this important morning meal. No surprise there. But the researchers also found that men who ate late at night—for instance, who got up for a midnight snack—were 55 percent more likely to have heart disease than men who didn't.

Why would late-night snacking lead to heart disease? There are many mechanisms, the most obvious of which is calories. People who snack at night tend to consume the same number of calories late at night as they would otherwise eat in the morning. Then they get up and eat more calories on top of that.[67]

Not long ago researchers at Brigham Young University asked 29 young men and women to avoid consuming any calories between 7 p.m. and 6 a.m. for two weeks. They also asked the participants to record every bite in a food journal.

Here's what happened. Skipping the nighttime snacks cut more than 200 calories from the daily total intake of each person. As a result, in just two weeks, without making any other lifestyle changes, the average study participant dropped just under a pound. When participants returned to their usual way of eating, however, they gained 1.3 pounds.[68]

But this is about more than just calories. Late-night snacking interrupts the fast that should take place between dinner and breakfast. Evidence is building that this fast is important. The body seems to need a daily digestive break so it can focus on repairing metabolic functions. There's some evidence that skipping this nightly fast can cause inflammation, blood sugar, blood fats, and oxidative stress all to rise.[69, 70]

Rx at a Glance

Make both your fast and breaking your fast mandatory. Try the following tricks:

* **Put a mental "closed" sign on your kitchen after dinner.** Or a real one. Try to completely shut down your eating by 8 or 9 p.m.

* **When you feel tempted to snack at night, go for a walk.** Drink water. Or do one of those activities that

you always say you will do when you have more time: read a book, clean, organize your closet.

* **Wake up and have a wholesome breakfast.** Steel-cut oats are a great option. I like to add a little almond or rice milk, a few raw walnuts, ground flax and chia seeds, and blueberries to supercharge the bowl with omega-3 fatty acids, fiber, and brain- and heart-friendly antioxidants. I always sprinkle spices such as apple pie, cinnamon, or pumpkin pie mix spices to increase the antioxidant power, too. If you are in a rush in the morning, a smoothie is a great option. Just make sure to use the 80-20 rule, making it mostly whole veggies, some fruits, and very little fruit juice. Add a nut butter (cashew, peanut, almond) for protein and energy.

YOUR FINAL FOOD PREP RX

Possibly the most important prescription I could ever share with you about heart-healthy eating is this: Just keep trying and you will never turn back. As with many things in life, healthy eating can be a "two steps forward, one step back" process. You might have a few days or a week during which you cook all your meals and manage to avoid junk foods. Then you have a day where you slip up. You fail to fire up the slow cooker. You go too long between meals, so hunger causes you to wolf everything down quickly.

And rather than mindfully enjoy that piece of dark chocolate, you mindlessly eat it while watching the news.

Then you go on to eat a whole host of foods while watching the news.

Then you are so disgusted with yourself that you think, "I'll never be able to follow a heart-healthy diet, so why bother?"

Do not go there.

No matter how much you think you've slipped up, just recommit to your main goal. If you need more motivation, ask your health care provider for a copy of your calcium score or some other test result. Tape it to your refrigerator. Let it shock you into action. Within as little as two weeks of your renewed commitment you will experience the enhanced energy, mental clarity, freedom from pain, and slimmer waistline that super-healthy eating offers everyone.

Chapter 8

Your Fitness Rx

You're about halfway through the book, and I like to think that I've captivated you. If you've been so engrossed that you've read from page 1 to page 147 in one sitting, it's probably time for you to stand up, and stretch.

Better yet, go for a short walk. Take the book with you and read as you go.

You probably think I'm joking. And I am, but only a little. Here's why: In the past several decades, researchers who study people and workplaces have concluded that our gluteus maximus, yes, our derriere, acts as if it has some type of aging sensor in it. *When we sit a lot, we activate that aging sensor and our risk for dying young from heart disease, diabetes, and other health problems increases.* Consider:

When Australian researchers asked more than 63,000 men about their chair time—how many minutes a day they spent sitting—and compared that data to their rates of chronic diseases (including heart disease, high blood pressure, and diabetes), they found that men who sat four or more hours a day were much more likely to have a chronic disease than men who sat less, and this was true regardless of their body weight or how much they exercised.[71]

148

Researchers from the Pennington Biomedical Research Center at Louisiana State University in Baton Rouge, Brigham and Women's Hospital, and Harvard Medical School have predicted that, if we'd all shrink our sitting time to fewer than three hours a day, our life expectancy would jump by two years.[72] Standing may be much more powerful for your health than most of the medicines you are taking!

People who spend more time being sedentary are 73 percent more likely to develop metabolic syndrome, a cluster of health problems that raise your risk factor for heart disease.[73]

It's long been shown that English bus drivers have far more heart disease than the conductors who ride on the very same double decker buses. What makes the difference? The bus drivers sit for 90 percent of their shifts, whereas the conductors stand, move around, and climb about 600 stairs a day as they take tickets from passengers on both levels of the bus.[74] Interestingly, Jeremy Morris, the epidemiologist who did this study in the 1940s and 1950s and who laid the groundwork for the aerobics movement of the 1980s, swam, pedaled a stationary bike, or walked every day. He lived to a ripe old age of 99.

You really should not take this news sitting down, but I understand that it's not easy to read while walking, especially if you don't own a treadmill desk. So it's okay to sit back down now if you'd like. Just, please, make sure to get back up and move once you finish this chapter.

WHY EXERCISE IS SO IMPORTANT

Getting fit will require more than simply breaking up with your favorite chair.

Standing isn't enough. You want to move with purpose. Yes, I'm talking about the e-word: exercise.

Physical activity is anything that makes you move your body and burn calories, such as climbing stairs, dancing, or playing sports. Aerobic exercise, such as walking, jogging, swimming, or biking, benefits your heart. Strength and stretching exercises are best for overall stamina and flexibility.

Exercise pushes your body out of its comfort zone, encouraging all of your muscles—including your heart—to grow stronger with every step. The importance of remaining as fit as a fiddle has been established in so many studies that it's difficult for me to pick just a few of my favorites. I hope these help to drive the point home. When researchers from Harvard, Stanford, and the London School of Economics pooled and analyzed the data from 16 different studies on hundreds of thousands of participants, they found that exercise was just as effective as most prescription drugs—and, in the case of stroke, more effective—at reducing deaths from heart disease.[75]

In a different study, researchers asked 4,183 male veterans to run on a treadmill while they were wearing sensors on their chests. The data from the sensors helped them to determine a measure called metabolic equivalent or MET. A MET is a common measurement used by exercise and cardiac specialists. One MET is the amount of energy burned by your body at rest. If you are doing an activity that burns twice that amount, you have reached 2 METS, five times the basal amount would be 5 METS, and so on. Average middle-aged people should be able to easily reach 9 to 10 METS on an exercise test.

Getting back to the researchers, they kept tabs on the men for seven years. For each 1 MET increase in exercise duration on the treadmill test, there was a 12 percent lower risk of dying during the seven years after. The most fit veterans had a 61 percent lower risk of dying—that's an astounding decrease of two-thirds!—compared to the least fit group.

As for the men who were out of shape at the beginning of the study and who worked on their fitness over the following seven years: They had a much lower risk of dying than those who remained in poor shape.[76]

It's pretty powerful data, and I hope it inspires you to grab your shoes and get moving.

Think of exercise, however you like to do it, as a powerful medi-

Do You Sit Too Much?

When I mention the dangers of sitting to my patients, many of them tell me that there's no way they sit four or more hours a day. Then I ask them a few questions.

- What do you do for work?
- How long does your job keep you seated each day?
- How long is your commute?
- How many hours of television do you watch in a given day?
- How many hours do you spend in front of a computer?
- What do you do for relaxation? Does it involve a chair?

Most are surprised to learn that they sit nine or more hours a day! And this is even true of some of my highly fit patients who love to run, cycle, swim, and do other forms of exercise. Chances are, you are sitting much more than you realize. So ask yourself the same questions. And consider that nine hours of sitting is more time in a chair than most of us spend asleep in our beds. Three hours is longer than it takes elite athletes to run the Boston Marathon! (And, surprisingly, you'll learn why the Boston Marathon might not be good for your heart in just a few pages.)

cine. Gym shoes, racquets, yoga mats, bicycles, dance floors, gardening tools, and barbells are real treatments of so many chronic conditions. Fitness activities can help you manage all of the following indicators of heart health:

Blood pressure. As I've said, exercise strengthens your cardiovascular system, allowing the heart to pump more blood with less effort. Some of this comes from training your leg and arm muscles to use oxygen more efficiently. Exercise also helps keep your arteries elastic and flexible, which allows them to expand to accommodate blood flow, again reducing pressure. Exercise is a stress reliever and helps control your weight. Both of these benefits may help lower your blood pressure.

And the benefit is a potent one. When researchers in Belgium pooled the results from more than 72 different studies on exercise and health, they found that exercise dropped blood pressure anywhere from two to seven points, and that the resistance inside the arteries dropped an average of seven percent.[77] That's similar to the effect of some blood pressure medicines, and getting fit might reduce your need for any prescription blood pressure medicines altogether. In one study, people who jogged two miles a day controlled their blood pressure so well that they were able to stop taking their medication.[78]

Blood sugar. Exercise makes your tissues more sensitive to insulin. That means cells throughout your body more easily absorb and burn blood sugar for energy. In fact, one study out of the University of Michigan found that exercise before eating regulated blood sugar almost as effectively as two different medicines commonly used to treat diabetes.[79] A recent study showed that a 15-minute walk after a meal kept blood sugar levels from spiking.[80] Exercise is a great way to delay or avoid diabetes mellitus, and it's also a great way to treat it. Patients with diabetes mellitus who exercise regularly also live longer than those who are sedentary.

Cholesterol. Exercise helps lower levels of triglycerides, those tiny packages of fat that float around in the bloodstream. It also stimulates enzyme systems in the muscles and liver that help to convert some unhealthy cholesterol into the potentially good HDL form. And it increases the size of the LDL and HDL particles, which makes them less likely to damage your arteries than the dense golf-ball-like small LDL particles.

Body weight. Because it burns calories, boosts metabolism, and encourages healthy eating, exercise can help you slim down. Whatever your weight, the more fit you are the lower your risk of dying. Without question, whatever style of eating you adopt, adding in regular and vigorous body movement will help you trim down.

Inflammation. I've told you how inflammation can cause so many chronic diseases, including heart disease. An analysis of

23 studies completed by Sunnybrook Research Institute and the University of Toronto found that levels of several markers of inflammation dropped after study participants started an exercise program.[81] By losing some inches around the waist you can lower the levels of irritant chemicals and mediators released from belly fat that transform your body into an inflammatory stew.

Blood clotting. Excessive blood clotting can lead to stroke, heart attack, and other cardiovascular problems. Regular exercise prevents clotting and clumping of blood cells.

Mood. Finally, exercise makes you happy. It creates physiological changes in the brain that lead to an increased sense of well-being, confidence, and an improved mood. Without a doubt your mind and your heart are closely connected.

Less than a third of adults exercise on a regular basis, and that's really a shame. Not only is exercise one of the more potent medicines you can take for your heart, it's also free. The benefits are near immediate: Your heart health will start to improve within days of starting a fitness plan. And people who are out of shape experience the most immediate benefits.

And it's not as hard as you might think. You can greatly improve your heart health and get fit without breaking a sweat. Sit less, move more. The prescriptions throughout these pages will help you accomplish just that.

Power Rx: Take a Five-Minute Walk

Do you want to know the top excuse I hear from patients when I suggest they get moving? It's this: I don't have enough time.

You know what? It's bogus, and I hope to prove it to you. You do have enough time. What you really need is motivation. Too often, people think of exercise in black or white categories: "thirty minutes" or "no minutes." In reality, any minutes of movement are better than none.

It's true that the American Heart Association recommends that we plan 150 minutes a week of moderate or 75 minutes a week of vigorous exercise. The goal of 30 minutes five times a week is an easy one, but it's not always possible.

What if you can't always make 150 minutes of exercise? Should you do none at all? No! Less activity than the AHA guideline is still of benefit. For one study, researchers followed the health habits and health outcomes of more than 400,000 people for eight years. When they crunched the data, they divided the group into inactive or low, medium, high, or very high activity levels. The low-activity group, who averaged only 15 minutes of exercise a

Ted's Journey to a Lasting Heart

Ted has a smile that invites you in as soon as you meet him. He has movie actor good looks and a soothing voice, too. Perhaps that's why I liked him the moment I met him.

When he first came to see me, he was in his early 40s and had already suffered a heart attack. Another physician had surgically placed several stents in his heart arteries, propping them open. Still, something was puzzling. Despite his stenting procedure, he still didn't feel comfortable. He didn't have true chest pain, called angina. But he just felt uncomfortable, especially whenever he bent his body in certain positions.

"Do you think the stents are flexing, causing the discomfort?" he asked.

I didn't think so, but I also couldn't come up with another explanation. His symptom had me stumped.

Ted had been living a generally healthy lifestyle up to his heart attack, but he also never said no to a slider and fries if he was with the guys. We discussed the basics of artery-friendly eating, stress management techniques, the importance of getting seven hours of good sleep, and regular exercise. After that appointment, he read half a dozen books on diet and stress, and he made major strides in changing his lifestyle.

But when he came back to see me, he pushed back a bit, telling me day, showed a 14 percent reduction in death compared with the completely inactive group. Groups that were more active showed even lower mortality.[82]

Got 15 minutes? Great.

Ten? That's good, too.

Even five minutes will bring you some benefits.

What's most important is this: Get started. You won't get any benefits if you continue to sit in your office chair, the driver's seat of your car, or your living room recliner.

that he didn't think he could ever fit exercise in. He felt bored whenever he used the elliptical or treadmill, and he questioned whether it was good to exercise the same muscles over and over. I had been increasing my own practice of yoga at the time, so I encouraged him to try a beginner's yoga class at a studio close to his home. They offered an early morning practice that would not interfere with his work commitments. I also suggested he read a yoga for beginners book, which he did.

Three months later, Ted was back. Now he had even more of a twinkle in his eye. He had really fallen in love with his yoga practice. He went on and on about how he felt that every part of his body was being used and strengthened, how the sweat was removing toxins from his body, how the community feeling of practicing mat to mat had offered him a sense of belonging, and how he had better self-control when his buddies ordered sliders and fries.

He reported with great joy that the vague pain over his heart that had followed him since his heart attack and stents was finally gone. When I examined him again six months later, his weight, blood pressure, and cholesterol were at all-time lows. He remained committed to the benefits of his yoga practice but smiled when he told me of one more unexpected benefit. He was dating one of his yoga instructors and was feeling as if a missing piece of his life was filled. We laughed and celebrated his growth.

Rx at a Glance

This is an easy one. Just get up and go. Remember:

* **Don't judge yourself.** If you are fatigued by the time you reach the mailbox, don't beat yourself up about it. Instead, congratulate yourself for putting in the effort.

* **Promise yourself that you'll do it again tomorrow.**

* **Focus on building a habit rather than on building fitness.** It's the everyday habit of movement that will eventually bring you the rewards of a fitter heart. It takes about 21 days to form a habit. So start with what you can handle, feel good about doing it every day, and don't stop.

Power Rx: Never Fast-Forward through a Commercial

For every two hours you spend in front of the TV, your risk of becoming obese jumps 23 percent and your risk of diabetes by 14 percent. This is true even if you exercise regularly. The more TV you watch—whether you are fit or not—the more time you spend sitting and the more likely you are to gain weight.[83]

The findings should give you pause. One tactic might be to cut down on TV time in general. If you did so, I'd applaud your efforts (and so would your heart).

But you don't have to go that far. You just need to learn how to multitask. James Levine, an endocrinologist with the Mayo Clinic, has spent his career studying the effects of exercise on health. He says that converting TV time to active time could allow some of us to shed 50 pounds a year! Marching in place during TV time? It could help you burn thousands of calories more over the course of 365 days.

If there are shows that I just have to watch, I will set up a TV in front of a treadmill, an elliptical, or a rowing machine. I will usually record the show and watch it early in the morning or later after work on replay. How about a few sit-ups or push-ups during commercials? How about a five-pound dumbbell lifted overhead 15 times with each arm for the 60-second break? I do that and make them calorie-burning commercials.

Another tactic: Pretend that the television is powered by your movement. Rather than sit as you watch, multitask. Stretch. Clean. March in place. You name it.

If that seems like too much, then, at the very least, don't ever take a commercial sitting down. Unless it's the Super Bowl, no one enjoys commercials. That's partially why some very smart person invented DVRs, so people could fast-forward through them. Don't do this. Instead, use every commercial as a cue to get up and move.

Rx at a Glance

For every 30 minutes of television programming, there are roughly eight minutes of commercials. Use this time wisely. Every time a commercial comes on:

* **Do calisthenics or stretches.**
* **March in place.**
* **Walk around the house.**
* **Complete a few active household chores.** Take out the trash, toss in a load of laundry, or change the sheets.

Power Rx: Practice Active Acts of Kindness

One way to motivate yourself to get in small, regular bouts of activity: Do them for someone else.

It's so important to move regularly throughout the day, and you've probably read advice telling you to take the stairs, park a little farther away, stand during phone calls, or do squats for five minutes every hour at work. It's good advice. In fact, it's advice that I hear myself telling people just about every day.

But here's my question: Are you doing any of it?

If you are, great. Give yourself a pat on the back.

If not, active acts of kindness may very well help you turn this around.

Rx at a Glance

Dedicate all of your small acts of exercise to the good of someone you love, to the happiness of a stranger, or to the good of society. Use these ideas for inspiration:

* **Return your shopping cart to the store** rather than leave it in the lot near your car. Do it as a favor to the kid whose job it is to go out and gather all the carts.

* **While you are out shoveling snow, shovel your neighbor's walkway, too.**

* **Offer to run an errand for someone you love,** and perform at least some of that errand on foot.

* **Walk into the bank rather than use the drive-thru,** just so you can tell the teller to have a "wonderful day."

* **Park farther away from your destination** so another driver, perhaps a little old lady or a mother with an infant, can have the closer space.

* **Get up and stand on the bus or the train** so someone else can have your seat.

* **Carry something heavy for someone else.**

* **Offer to put someone's bag in the overhead compartment on an airplane.**

Power Rx: De-motorvate Your Life

At the turn of the millennium, seven male actors answered help wanted ads from a theme park in Australia called "Old Sydney Town." A tribute to the eighteenth and early nineteenth centuries, the town was designed exactly as the city of Sydney looked in 1803. There were authentically reconstructed buildings, soldiers on parade, cannons, duels, and even convict rebellions.

What wasn't there: any device that required batteries or electricity, because such things had not yet been invented in the early 1800s.

Nor were there cars.

Once on the job, the actors agreed to have researchers fit them with triaxial accelerometers to measure their activity levels. For comparison, they used the same devices to measure the activity levels of seven office workers.

The results were startling. The actors ended up moving around 60 percent more than the office workers, walking up to nine miles more every single day![84]

As many experiments by James Levine, an endocrinologist with the Mayo Clinic, have found, time-saving devices save more than time. They also save calories. Consider how many fewer calories you burn when you:

* Use a dishwasher rather than wash dishes by hand: half a calorie less per minute.

* Drive to work rather than walk: 2.6 fewer calories per minute walked.

* Use the elevator rather than take the steps: 3 fewer calories per minute.

When Levine added all of the time-saving devices up, he concluded that they cause the average person to save 111 calories a day. Over time, that adds up to 10 extra pounds a year. It would take you 45 minutes of steady walking every single day to burn off those calories saved by time-saving devices, Levine predicts.[85]

Rx at a Glance

Whenever possible, try not to motor your way through life. Do it in the name of your heart. Do it for your weight, and do it for the environment. Here are a few ideas to get you started. Use:

* **A push mower** instead of a riding one, and a manual one instead of a gas- or electric-powered one.
* **A broom or a rake** instead of a leaf blower.
* **The sink** instead of the dishwasher.
* **The clothesline** instead of the clothes dryer.
* **A broom or a mop** instead of the vacuum.
* **Your body** instead of a remote control.
* **Your elbow grease** instead of an electric mixer.
* **Your hands** instead of a bread maker.
* **Your feet** instead of a golf cart.

Power Rx: Don't Take Waiting Sitting Down

We hate to wait, and executives from the Houston airport have proof. Several years ago, in response to complaints from passengers about having to wait for their bags at baggage claim, the airport did something about it. It hired more baggage handlers, which slashed the average wait to just eight minutes.

You'd think the complaints would've stopped. They didn't. People complained just as much as ever. When executives studied the matter, they realized that it only took passengers a minute to walk to baggage claim, so three-quarters of their time between the plane and the car was spent waiting.

What the executives did next was near genius, in my opinion. They moved the airport gates away from the main terminal so passengers would have to walk six times longer to get to baggage claim. Once they got there, they only had to wait a minute or two for their bags. Sometimes they didn't have to wait at all.

The complaints dropped to almost zero.

We stand and wait a lot: at the grocery store, at the bank, at the post office, at the ATM, at amusement parks, and, yes, at baggage claims.

And that's the waiting that we do standing. A lot of it we take sitting down. Consider what you do while waiting in, um, a waiting room? Or what you do during the average 10 to 20 minutes each of us spends on hold on the telephone each week?

Rx at a Glance

Sure, people in the waiting room might look askance if you spend your time marching in place, but you really don't have to take many of these situations sitting down. I try to move or stand as much as possible. When I'm at morning meetings or conferences, for instance, I quietly move to the back of the auditorium and I pace back and forth as I listen. Use these ideas whenever you find yourself waiting:

* **March in place.**
* **Try some calisthenics.**
* **Do a few laps around the house.**
* **Climb a flight of stairs.**
* **Try a few stretches.**
* **Do a few yoga sun salutations.**
* **Do burpees** (a Marine-style exercise that involves jumping down to the floor, doing a push-up, jumping back up to do a jumping jack, and repeating) or jumping jacks.
* **Straighten up the house.**

* **Pull a few weeds from the garden.**
* **Or at least stand.**

Power Rx: Get a Pedometer

I've mentioned a physician at the Mayo Clinic, Dr. James Levine, already. He has pioneered many forms of workplace and daily activities and he calls these non-exercise activity thermogenesis (NEAT).

Those big words mean you are not gearing up in your sweat suit and sneakers, but you are building calorie-burning into your day at a frequent but low level. Dr. Levine feels that NEAT is actually more important than your gym time, which goes back to the idea that butt time is bad time. In fact, studies show people who regularly go to the gym for workouts but sit the rest of the day at their workplace fare little better than those who don't exercise at all.

That is not an excuse not to go to the gym, but the best approach is the gym plus NEAT.

Rx at a Glance

The easiest way to stay focused on NEAT is to wear a pedometer and measure how many steps a day you are taking. These are available to clip on your waist for $25, as applications to your smartphone, or as high-tech pocket or wrist digital devices for around $100. There are sites that track your steps, and 10,000 steps a day is often a goal. It is important not to be frustrated if you start to use a pedometer and find you are recording well under 5,000 steps. Set a goal to increase by perhaps 500 steps a day for a week, then jump it up again to the next level.

How are you going to increase your NEAT using a pedometer? New habits will get you there:

* **Park as far as possible from the entrance to work.** I do this every day, enjoying a 10-minute walk each morning and each evening. I also get fewer marks on my car because the farther parking spaces also happen to be the least crowded and, consequently, most spacious.

* **Take the stairs up or down one or two flights routinely if you can.**

* **Spend half of your lunch hour walking.**

* **Ask your employer to mark walking paths** that are safe and well lit or organize walking clubs.

* **Propose a walking meeting** if you don't require access to a computer during the meeting. This not only adds NEAT to your day (and your colleagues'), but also enhances creativity, particularly if you can walk outside.

* **Walk after dinner.** Doing so does more than help you sneak in some extra movement. As I mentioned earlier, a post-meal walk goes a long way to helping your body to manage blood sugar. This is especially true if you went a bit too heavy on dessert. Plus it's a nice ritual that can bring you closer to family members as well as help you mentally transition out of eating and into the rest of the evening.

* **Get off two bus stops earlier** than your destination.

* **Park one block away** from where you want to go.

* **Take a short walk** whenever you arrive at a destination a little early.

* **Keep walking shoes in your car or at work** so you can go for a quick walk whenever you need to energize your brain.

* **Get a dog.** They can be the best walking partners—and can also help you reduce stress, as you'll learn in Chapter 9.

* **Play actively with your kids.** Play tag, flag football, hide and seek, Twister, or even mini golf.

* **Never drive through a drive-thru.** You're not going to fast food establishments at all, but you'll encounter drive-thrus at the bank, the pharmacy, and even the liquor store. Always park and get out of your car.

* **Walk around the terminal** as you wait in the airport and avoid the moving sidewalks. Many airports offer lockers you can rent and store your luggage in as you walk.

Power Rx: Stand Whenever Possible

Although standing may not register steps on a pedometer, the data on sitting time being bad for your health is quite strong and growing all the time. Even if you can't actually walk, standing is still, by far, one better than sitting.

I am known by a lot of nicknames: the vegan cardiologist, the yoga cardiologist, the holistic cardiologist, and so on. But I am proudest of one title in particular: the standing cardiologist. I stand whenever I can. When I am seeing patients, I stand for most of the consult. Then, when I'm doing record keeping and notations afterward, I use a higher counter so I can stand as I dictate. Hospitals are NOT healthy places. We physicians are asked to attend meeting after meeting. Of course, the doughnuts and muffins are at the back of every single one of those meetings, breaking every food rule. Of more concern, 50 or 100 cardiac specialists will gather and not move for the whole 30, 60, or 90 minutes—and these are all people who are well aware of the research.

I take the stairs whenever possible. In fact, at several of the hospitals where I work, we have placed signs announcing it as a StairWELL, and I often meet other walkers dedicated to their health on their way up or down.

At conferences and meetings, I choose seats in the back or side of auditoriums and conference rooms and quickly move out of my chair to stand, pace, and stretch. A few eyebrows go up, but I know that more are wondering why they are not doing that, too. I also feel that my mind is sharper by standing and moving and I participate in the conversation more fully when I am working on my fitness and not my seated fatness. I would urge you to start a trend wherever you have meetings to get up and work standing. Move it or lose it.

Rx at a Glance

How do you do it? Use this advice:

* **When you make phone calls, stand as much as you can.**

* **Prop your computer up to waist height,** so you can stand while working. I wrote this chapter, in fact, while I was standing with the laptop on a high kitchen counter or while walking on my treadmill desk.

* **Stand or roam at the side or back of the room** when you are at a presentation, lecture, or performance, if appropriate.

* **At a minimum, take a five- to 10-minute break hourly** to stand, stretch, and move as much as possible.

Power Rx: If You Miss a Week, Don't Throw in the Towel

There are two critical times that many people fall off the exercise wagon: after a really busy period at work and after a vacation.

What happens is that they skip one workout and then another and then another. Soon they've gone a week or two without exercise and they think, "Why bother? I've lost everything I've gained."

But this isn't true at all. You haven't lost everything. In fact, you probably haven't lost much at all. Duke researchers proved this when they put 183 out-of-shape, overweight men and women who were at risk for developing heart disease through the paces of an eight-month-long exercise plan. Once they got everyone in shape, they wanted to see what would happen if everyone blew off their workouts. So they asked all the study participants to take two weeks off. All the while the researchers measured changes in their blood cholesterol and other markers of heart health.

Even after a two-week break, study participants still maintained some benefits. They had not gone back to day one. In particular, their triglycerides remained low and HDL cholesterol remained high.[86] It takes five to six weeks of totally stopping exercise for the number of healthy mitochondria in your muscles to fall back to baseline. They will increase back to healthier and increased numbers again if you get back to moving.

Rx at a Glance

Recommit yourself to exercise as soon as you can, whenever you can. Don't fall prey to the excuse: "I've lost everything." When you recommit:

* **Go easy on yourself.** Cut back on your intensity and duration. Ease yourself back into the swing of things.

* **Congratulate yourself** for doing something—anything—to stop the slide back into inactivity.

* **Commit with a friend or relative** to walk or bike together and promise each other not to let the other person down.

Power Rx: Take Vitamin Y (Try Yoga)

I couldn't write a chapter about fitness without taking a moment to promote one of my favorite fitness pursuits.

I started practicing yoga more than 10 years ago and I felt very out of my element. I hung in the back of the room next to a wall. Ashtanga what? Vinyasa who? Kundalini where? Namaste, or was it namastea or namastomato?

But the group setting, the music, and the patience of instructors were all helpful.

Now I have come to appreciate how efficient yoga is. It's like a four-for-one exercise. Most people don't realize that certain types of yoga (especially hot yoga and continuous-flowing movement sequences) count as cardio. I have worn my heart rate monitor during classes and my pulse gets as high as it does when I am running on the treadmill. Yoga also strengthens your muscles, so it counts as weight training, too. Of course, it gets you flexible. Finally, the emphasis on breath work and the power of your thoughts makes it a moving meditation.

Some poses—such as Tree and Dancer's Pose—also improve your balance, preventing falls. I keep telling myself that when I fall out of a balancing pose (always), I am getting stronger.

Here are three more reasons to give it a try:

A more consistent heart rate. One of the most important ways yoga can benefit your cardiovascular health is through heart rate variability (HRV). The term HRV reflects the ability of the heart rate to change beat to beat. If you're healthy and you breathe in deeply, your heart rate will speed up; if you exhale deeply, the opposite will occur. These rapid changes occur predominantly due to the influence of the parasympathetic nervous system (PNS). This healthy response is counterbalanced by the sympathetic nervous system (SNS), which releases adrenaline, a stress hormone. When the PNS predominates, HRV is high during deep breathing, stress is reduced, and health is promoted. The SNS predominates during stress, and in sufferers of diseases like diabetes mellitus, heart disease, kidney failure, and other conditions.

There are nearly 900 research studies measuring HRV in humans, both in healthy and disease states. In survivors of heart attacks, diabetic patients, COPD patients, people with congestive heart failure, in smokers, and even in the general population, these studies have shown that low HRV leads to loss of cardiac nervous system PNS/SNS balance and an increased risk of dying suddenly. Yikes, that's a serious outcome! As an example of what a low HRV looks like, I've seen patients with a resting heart rate of 100 that won't vary at all during deep breathing. This is worrisome to me.

HRV has been measured in people both before and after practicing various styles of yoga for a given period. For example, following eight weeks of Hatha yoga, nine of 12 subjects showed a significant increase in HRV.[87] In another study, 45 pregnant women participating in yoga for an hour a day were compared to the same number who did not attend the classes. Stress was reduced only in the yoga group, and by the thity-sixth week of practice, HRV increased by 150 percent.[88]

Less atrial fibrillation. Atrial fibrillation is the most common cardiac rhythm disturbance. Caused by high blood pressure, leaky heart valves, and several other factors, it leads to frequent office and hospital visits, costing millions (if not billions) of health care dollars. It's an unpredictable disorder of the heart rhythm and can interfere with work, vacations, and family gatherings. Recently patients with intermittent atrial fibrillation were studied for three months as a baseline and then followed for three more months while practicing yoga twice a week for 60 minutes. During the three months of yoga practice, episodes of atrial fibrillation dropped in frequency, and patients rated their quality of life as better, too. There were also decreases in blood pressure and resting heart rate.[89]

Lower blood pressure. Recently 50 patients with high blood pressure participated in a yoga practice for 15 days, lasting two hours each session. Cardiac function was assessed before and after this training. After practicing yoga for two weeks, patients experienced significantly reduced resting heart rates and systolic and diastolic blood pressures. A comparison group that did not do the training did not experience these benefits.[90]

Rx at a Glance

There are yoga rooms that are kept at comfortable temperatures, ones that are kept hot, and then the ultra-hot classes that are not for the beginner. Keep in mind:

* **Start with a beginner's class in a room at a comfortable temperature.** This might even be with a DVD you try at home, and there are many excellent choices. Classes where you remain in your chair are suited for new students of all ages and health levels. Consider a private lesson one to two times to get started without fear.

* **Pain is not gain.** Yoga should not hurt. If you are bending something and it is giving you a painful message, stop and readjust your body.

* **Whenever you need to, take a break in Child's Pose.** You are not competing with the person on the next mat. If you are patient with yourself, you will come to see the benefits of a regular practice even if you can't put your heel behind your head.

* **Do it once a week or every day.** Even practiced once a week, even for only 15 to 20 minutes, yoga offers flexibility, mental focus, and relaxation. I have friends who have avoided back surgery by doing a gentle home yoga flow 10 minutes twice a day. If you enjoy it, yoga can be practiced daily for 30 to 60 minutes, as the options are almost limitless.

Power Rx: Move in the Morning

The morning is the best time to fit in a workout and here's why: It puts your workout in the number one position on your to-do list.

When you exercise later in the day, dozens of obstacles and excuses are likely to come up, ranging from "I'm too hungry" to "Oh, way too busy" to "I'm just too tired." When you roll out of bed and get moving first thing, those excuses don't have a chance to derail your motivation. You don't even have a chance to feel hungry if you start moving right away. (Note: Although it's usually best to exercise on an empty stomach, a small snack such as piece of fruit or a glass of vegetable juice can quell hunger and perk you up.) And that initial tiredness will soon give way to total body clarity and energy.

There's also some evidence that a morning workout can undo some of the metabolic damage of whatever fatty, high-sugar foods you might have consumed the night before.[91]

Rx at a Glance

Do your workout in the morning. I fit some kind of workout into my life five or six days a week, on average, and almost all of them are early morning workouts. I try to get in bed at a reasonable hour so the early morning wake-up alarm isn't met by a groan and the snooze button. I find that attending a gym and participating in a group fitness class like spinning, aerobics, or yoga motivates me to show up because others expect me there. If I skip these classes for a few days, texts start to come in either inquiring about my well-being or chastising me for being a lazy old man! It is helpful.

There are, of course, many cold and dark winter nights in Detroit when the thought of getting in a cold car at 4:30 a.m., a habit I am famous for in town, to reach the health club for a 5:00 a.m. group fitness class does not sound exciting. On those days, I don't sleep in. Rather, I head to the basement. If time is short I will warm up on a treadmill with 20 minutes of fast walking and then do a 15-minute high-intensity Tabata routine (see page 173) that has my heart rate reaching high levels intermittently. I either use a rowing machine or floor exercise to do this.

Use this advice:

* **Go to bed earlier, and get up earlier, too.** Often the last half hour before bed is wasted time. We use it to watch TV or surf Facebook. Delete that wasted time from your life so you wake refreshed and ready to move.

* **Try exercising on an empty stomach.** If you feel okay, great. If you don't, consider eating a small amount of easily digestible food, such as a banana, before you head out.

* **Agree to meet someone.** This will ensure you actually get out of bed rather than hit the snooze button.

Another tip I find helpful: If I can't fit in exercise, I commit myself to eating even healthier that day, making every bite fresher, more organic, and more colorful.

Power Rx: Invest $10 a Month in Movement

Many costs have gone up in recent years, but a gym membership is not one of them. In fact, most cost less than ever before.

It wasn't that long ago when a $30-a-month membership was considered a bargain. Today in some parts of the country some popular chains offer memberships for a third of that: a mere $10 a month.

By joining a gym, you'll have access to weights, cardio machines, stretch bands, Pilates machines, Swiss balls, yoga mats, kettlebells, and other types of equipment. You might also be able to take classes and get advice from staff trainers. And the indoor environment gives you somewhere to work out when it's too hot, too humid, too cold, too icy, too rainy, too polluted, or just too dreary to exercise outdoors. It's not a requirement to getting your fitness fix, but a gym certainly helps keep you consistent.

Rx at a Glance

When joining a gym, consider:

* **Location.** The closer it is to home or work, the more likely you'll use it.
* **The staff.** If you've never exercised before, you'll benefit from a knowledgeable staff. Some gyms offer one free personal training session with your membership.
* **The equipment.** Gyms with pools and racquetball courts generally cost more than gyms without them.
* **Child care.** Some offer it. Others don't.

If you have never exercised, think about hiring a personal trainer for at least a few sessions. Let him or her know of any medical problems you have. If you have a known heart condition, a phone call to your health care provider before exercise might be a good idea. No matter what, gym or basement, work or backyard, move it or lose it. That includes your heart, your memory, and your health.

Power Rx: Stay out of Your Comfort Zone

No, I'm not talking about the comfort zone on the couch. I'm talking about the one during exercise, when you are so used to doing a particular movement that you zone out and go through the motions.

Research shows that we need more than one type of exercise: stretching to maintain flexibility, strengthening, balance exercises, and cardio. You may know weight lifters who couldn't touch their toes for $100, runners who never do a push-up, people who lift a leg and fall, and so on. Rotating exercises to balance the body provides the best results.

Our bodies adapt quickly to exercise, giving us declining results over time. And so do our minds. When we go through the motions, we feel bored. When we feel bored, we don't work as hard.

And we're also a lot less likely to keep it up.

Rx at a Glance

Variety is important. Continually mix it up by:

* **Rotating between heart-rate thumping cardio, weight training, and flexibility activities.** Balance is the best approach.
* **Trying new classes and exercises.** Many gyms have now branched out and are offering activities previously seen only in specialty fitness centers. These include yoga, tai-chi and other martial arts, Pilates, Zumba, and barre classes.
* **Going harder on some days and easier on others.** For instance, you might try to do just six lifts of very heavy weights on some days, but more like 12 or even 15 lifts of lighter weights on others. Similarly, if you are into yoga (see the Power Rx on page 167), your easy day might be a restorative class, whereas the harder day could be the flow yoga. It is not essential to push to the maximum at every workout, and even quiet movements like chair yoga, tai chi, and regular walking have tremendous benefits that can be woven into a regular exercise plan.

Power Rx: Go Hard for 20 Seconds

A growing body of scientific support is developing for a type of training called high-intensity interval training. These workouts were developed nearly 20 years ago in Japan by Dr. Izumi Tabata for Olympic athletes and are often called Tabata workouts.

His protocol is 20 seconds of the most intense exercise you can do, followed by 10 seconds of rest, repeated eight times. The entire workout is four minutes long. In research done by Dr. Tabata, when athletes doing these workouts four times a week were compared to others doing steady endurance workouts five times a week for much longer periods of time, there were equal gains. And it took just four minutes.[92] They can be done on a treadmill, elliptical, or rowing machine, but I would recommend a medical checkup before beginning these challenging activities.

Another professor, Martin Gibala at McMaster University in Hamilton, Ontario, has shown similar findings with a slightly different program.[93] This involves a three-minute warm-up, followed by 60 seconds of intense exercise, followed by 75 seconds of cool-down, repeated eight to 12 times. A final cool-down of five minutes is then performed.

Other options include 60 seconds on and off as well as 60 seconds on and 30 off. In general, the more time you spend exercising and the less time you spend resting, the better your fitness results.

These types of intense workouts are clearly not for everybody. Anyone with heart or orthopedic issues or multiple medical problems should discuss them with a medical professional first and may want to consider working with a trainer when first trying an interval workout.

Rx at a Glance

If you are thinking about doing this form of exercise, all you really need—in its simplest form—is your body. If you have a jump rope, give yourself extra credit. Here's how to get started:

* **Read about Drs. Tabata and Gibala on the Internet.** There are many sites that will give you background, inspiration, and ideas.

* **Download the Tabata app onto your phone.** It will count down your segments for you, sounding an

alarm whenever it's time to rest or restart a segment. In lieu of the app, you can also use a stopwatch.

* **Consider meeting friends and taking turns designing Tabata-style workouts.** This can be a fun social activity that gets you all fit. Each session, allow one person to be in charge of keeping track of the time.

* **Listen to your body.** If you are experiencing pain or significant shortness of breath during these workouts, stop and discuss your symptoms with your physician.

If it feels good, go for it. High intensity is built into our systems. We used to have to run from saber-toothed tigers at full speed. Now we are learning that same intensity trains our body quickly.

Power Rx: Walk While You Work

As I wrote this chapter, when I didn't have my laptop propped on a kitchen counter, I had it on an elevated desk that I purchased on the Internet. That allowed me to walk on a treadmill at 1.5 to 2.0 miles per hour as I typed. At this speed it is possible to search the web, type, read, and text on my phone.

I can do all of this while wearing a suit. That's because I'm walking slowly enough that I never break a sweat. I can rush back to work and not have to worry about someone asking me why beads of perspiration are on my brow.

At the same time, however, I am not activating those "aging sensors" in my rear.

I have spent thousands of hours over the years reading my medical journals in this manner.

Rx at a Glance

Invented by Dr. James Levine many years ago, treadmill desks have been shown to more than double your calorie burn during the workday, incinerating 100 more calories for every hour spent on the job. If you are currently obese, this one change could help you shed 44 to 66 pounds in a year's time, according to Levine's research.[94]

Although exotic and expensive when he introduced them over 10 years ago, they have come down in price a lot, and the desk can be built or bought for a few hundred dollars or less if you have a treadmill. The combined desk/treadmill units designed for workplaces are around $1,000. Many offices have installed one or several; they can be quite popular. Ask your office to consider one, or think about getting one at home if you do a lot of paperwork, reading, or phone calls. It might seem expensive at first, but whatever amount you spend, think how much bypass surgery, stents, and medications cost. I guarantee the treadmill desk is cheaper!

Power Rx: Run Long Distances like a Turtle

In the year 490 BCE, the fittest runner in Greece, Phiddipides, ran 26 miles from Marathon to Athens, to announce a great victory over the Persians. After declaring the news, he dropped dead.

Now, 2,500 years later, we might finally understand why. We might call it the Phiddipides effect.

Data is emerging that question whether repeated long-distance endurance events—ranging from marathons to triathlons—are good for the heart. Many studies have examined runners just after they've completed a marathon (26.2-mile run), finding that the events strain the heart for hours to days afterward. These studies have found that more than half of distance runners leak a protein in the blood called troponin. When we detect this protein in the blood of people who show up at the ER with chest pain, we know they are having a heart attack. If this isn't disturbing enough, echocardiograms (ultrasound examinations of the heart) and heart MRI scans have been done on runners immediately after a marathon and again a week or two later. The scans right after a marathon often show that a part of the heart called the right ventricle is acutely enlarged at the end of a marathon. While this returns to normal eventually, it's trouble because scar tissue might ultimately develop if one runs repeated marathons. This could make the scarring permanent, thickening heart tissue and leading to serious rhythm problems. MRI heart scans have also found chronic scarring of the heart in these distance runners, and one study found that nearly 15 percent of athletes who participated in multiple endurance events had these scars.[95]

Another piece of data suggests that calcium deposits in arteries of regular long-distance runners are actually more advanced than in people who exercise far less. Finally, a rhythm problem of the heart called atrial fibrillation is often found as much as four to five times more often in the marathon runners than in controls.

The city of Copenhagen has been performing a heart follow-up study on thousands of citizens living there. The amount and intensity of exercise has been studied and follow-up death rates have been measured for over two decades now. The work from that city describes a U-shaped curve. Inactive people have the highest mortality, moderate exercisers had a much lower mortality, and those who are pushing the envelope with frequent, fast, and long endurance exercises have a lower mortality than the couch potatoes, but a higher mortality than the moderate exercisers.

Rx at a Glance

It may turn out, after all, that the turtle was right—slow and steady does win the race. Based on this data, researchers have concluded that the "sweet spot" of running is a medium pace, no more than three times a week, and less than 2.5 hours total per week. If you burn to do an ultra-endurance event, use these pointers:

* **Do it at a young age and train properly.** That means slowly build up your fitness, adding no more than 10 percent to your weekly or daily miles at any one time.

* **Consider cross-training, limiting your pace and distance, and mixing walking and running.**

* **Space your endurance events many months apart.** No one is sure about the right span of time between events at the moment. If you do many events, consider cutting out every other one.

* **Eat an anti-inflammatory, plant-based diet while training to lower injury and promote recovery.** This is a good diet to follow 24/7, but it's more important than ever if you are training for an endurance event.

YOUR FINAL FITNESS RX

I hope this chapter has made you look differently at that over-stuffed Lazy Boy sitting in front of your big-screen TV. It's starting to look a lot more like the electric chair than a place to relax, isn't it?

If so, good.

Indeed, if there were a single pill that offered all the benefits that exercise does, it would be a blockbuster seller. If we all made it our goal to walk to the pharmacy to pick up our prescriptions, we might not need our prescriptions anymore!

Once you understand that prolonged sitting is a life-robbing activity and running repeated marathons is neither necessary nor clearly protective for the heart, you can take an approach to movement that is much like eating. If you understand some simple rules and strategies, and you are intent on aging without chronic diseases, you can figure out a program that works for you. The main thing is to aim to move more and sit less every day.

In fact, posting that on your computer or desk to remind you would be a good start.

Chapter 9

Your Emotional Health Rx

The text on my phone was from an emergency room physician. It read: "A lady with a friggin' big heart attack!" Next came a picture of the ECG (yes, cell phones can be great medical communication tools). I looked at the page and saw that this patient had huge abnormalities on her ECG, a sign often called "tombstone elevation." It was an indication of a major heart attack. I knew she was in trouble.

"Yes, that's a big one," I thought.

As you might expect, I rushed to the hospital. Would I be able to do anything to save her? Even if I could open her totally blocked artery with an emergency stent, would her life forever be limited by a weakened heart muscle, one that caused her to feel fatigued while doing the simplest of tasks? Would she ever be able to again experience simple pleasures such as playing with her grandchildren? I didn't know.

When I walked into the ER, I was surprised to see a nicely dressed woman sobbing quietly. I did a double take. Had I walked into the wrong room? Usually heart attack patients are squirming and writhing in pain, and they look like they want relief right away.

This patient didn't seem to be in much distress. As the team rushed her to the heart catheterization room, I had a chance to ask her a few questions. I learned that she had been at an AA meeting with her daughter, who was in recovery. During the meeting, her first, she felt she'd failed as a mother, and her shame and stress were intense. She began to feel horrible chest pressure.

In the next 10 minutes, I performed an angiogram that showed that she had normal heart arteries. None of them was clogged. I saw no blood clots. Blood was flowing through them without obstruction.

Her heart, however, was another matter. It looked like it had been run over by a semi. A large portion of it was not beating at all.

Fortunately, with proper medication, nutrition, and vitamins, she completely recovered her heart strength within four weeks and is doing fine now, months later. She is playing with her grandchildren, too.

You might wonder: How could my patient have sustained that much damage to her heart if her arteries were perfectly healthy?

It's called Broken Heart Syndrome. It got its name because it was first diagnosed in people who were grieving the loss of a loved one. The first patients to be diagnosed with it experienced their first chest pains during a funeral or just after learning of a divorce. Now we know that *any type of intense stress can bring it on, whether it's a car accident, a job loss, a mugging, or something else.* It often manifests in women more than men, and it's one example of the many ways our emotional well-being influences the well-being of our hearts.

HOW NEGATIVITY BREAKS YOUR HEART

In the 1950s we developed a theory that all heart attacks were caused by one problem: Eat too many fat- and cholesterol-laden foods and the cholesterol in your blood will build up, we thought. Once cholesterol built up, the arteries would narrow. When arteries narrowed, not as much blood could flow. Eventually, if arteries narrowed enough, the heart was starved of blood. End result: a heart attack.

We now know, as I mentioned in Chapter 2, that this is an overly simplistic understanding of the progression of heart disease. But several decades ago, it was considered the status quo.

Then, in the early to mid-1950s, two free-spirited and perceptive cardiologists in San Francisco noticed something strange: Many of their patients were consuming healthy diets. Yet they still had heart disease.

The cardiologists, Meyer Friedman and R. H. Rosenman, wondered why.

They also wondered something else: Why were the chairs in their waiting room frayed along the front edges rather than around the back areas? When they casually paid attention to what was going on in their waiting room, they noticed that their heart patients tended to sit on the edges of their seats. They also tended to leap up frequently, often to ask a question like, "How much longer do I have to wait?"

This intrigued Dr. Friedman, possibly because he was as high-strung and tense as many of the patients he treated. He was driven, impatient, and often finished other people's sentences for them or rushed them along with a "yup, yup, come to the point." So he began observing 40 accountants to see what happened to their cholesterol levels during tax season. In March their cholesterol levels went up. After tax season ended, cholesterol levels dropped.

In the 1970s Dr. Friedman introduced two new terms, "type A" and "type B." People who were type A were impatient and chronically stressed, and his research indicated that type A people had an increased risk of heart disease and heart attacks.

His observation started a wave of research into the effects of stress on the heart. We now know that any type of chronic negativity stresses the heart.

Any type of stress—whether it be chronic or acute—triggers the nervous system to unleash adrenaline, cortisol, and other so-called "stress hormones." If you're under a great deal of stress—for instance, when you learn a loved one was just killed in a car accident—this sudden wave of stress hormones can stun the heart, preventing it from effectively pumping blood and bringing on the symptoms of a heart attack.

When you are under chronic stress, the mechanism is slightly different. The body's immune system fights stress as it would fight a disease or infection. In response to stress, the immune system produces cortisol, adrenaline, and inflammatory proteins called cytokines, including interleukin-6. As I've mentioned, over time this chronic inflammation leads to arteriosclerosis (hardening of the arteries) and heart disease.

Let's take a look at how different types of negativity raise your risk:

Stress. Even if you are healthy in every other way—you exercise and you eat a truckload of vegetables—stress can still affect your heart. In a study from the Netherlands, scientists studied three-centimeter-long hair samples from 238 senior citizens and tested them for the presence of the stress hormone cortisol. (Much as each ring of a tree equals a year in time, each centimeter of hair includes roughly a month of aging information.) People with high levels of this stress hormone were more likely to have a history of heart disease, stroke, and diabetes than people with low levels.[96] People with a high amount of perceived stress were also at a 27 percent increased risk for heart disease, and levels of the bad LDL cholesterol tended to be as much as 50 mg/dL higher. Their blood pressure was also an average 2.7/1.4 mmHg more than people with low stress. When added up, that's the health equivalent of smoking five cigarettes per day![97]

Depression. Middle-aged women who are depressed have double the risk of having a stroke as those who aren't, and depressed stroke survivors have triple the risk of death as non-depressed stroke survivors.[98] Like stress, depression seems to undo the positive effects of healthy lifestyle choices such as exercise. People who are physically active tend to have lower levels of an inflammatory protein in their blood called C-reactive protein (CRP). But depressed people who are fit experience no such benefit.[99]

Depression might lead to heart disease the same way stress does, by changing the body's hormonal chemistry for the worse. There is some preliminary but provocative data that shows inflammatory markers in the blood (such as interleukin-6, a pro-inflammatory chemical) are elevated in people who are depressed. People who are depressed also tend to practice other unhealthy behaviors. They eat poorly and tend to be sedentary, and they are less likely to follow doctor's orders.

Anxiety. Heart disease patients who suffer from anxiety have twice the risk of death as those who don't have anxiety. And patients with anxiety and depression have triple the risk of death.[100]

These aren't the only types of negativity that can hurt your heart. Others include: low self-esteem, loneliness, anger, hostility, and hopelessness.

HOW POSITIVE EMOTIONS CAN HEAL

Positive emotions are like a healing balm. They obliterate the effects of stress, and they lead to vitality and well-being.

We now know that our hearts (and our guts) are miniature brains, complete with their own supply of neurons (nerve cells) that transmit signals from the heart to the brain. The heart can also release substances that stimulate the release of oxytocin, the love hormone. This hormone boosts our well-being and triggers us to bond with others. A long, tight hug releases oxytocin and strengthens your heart health.

Our emotions can also influence the heart. When we are aroused by passion or anger, our hearts beat more quickly. When we feel calm, the heart rate slows.

You might think, "Well, that's nice, but it's not as if I can force myself to feel happy!" That's not completely true. Sure, telling yourself, "Feel happy! Feel happy! Feel happy!" probably isn't going to work. But that doesn't mean that positive emotions like happiness, joy, and inner peace are not within your control. You can take steps to make over your mind from negative to positive. Our habits and daily activities—from breathing to meditation to sleep—have a proven impact on our emotional well-being. Even things that we rarely think of as being important—such as human touch, pets, and treatments such as acupuncture—can have a dramatic impact on mood, emotional well-being, the quality of our sleep, and our ability to relax.

And it doesn't take very long at all to experience dramatic results. As you'll soon find, within just five minutes, you can feel significantly better!

Power Rx: Laugh at Least Once a Day

How about a good old belly laugh? Can mirth, giggling, and playfulness really help the heart?

Indeed they can.

When researchers compared blood flow in people watching a stressful movie *(Saving Private Ryan)* compared to people watching comedy like *Saturday Night Live,* they documented a 35 percent reduction in blood flow during the stressful movie and a 22 percent increase in circulation in those laughing and enjoying themselves.[101]

This increase in blood flow is on par with what is seen with some of the most established prescription medications. And there are no side effects . . . except maybe snorting!

This experiment was repeated on patients in Japan with similar results. It's likely that laughter releases endorphins (happy chemicals) from the brain, and these hormones result in arteries dilating and resisting the clotting of blood.

Rx at a Glance

Make it your goal to laugh at least once a day, using the following ideas as inspiration:

* Watch comedies instead of tragedies.

* Constantly be on the lookout for reasons to laugh at yourself rather than get angry with yourself or others.

* Take turns telling funny stories or jokes with family members.

Power Rx: Drop Blood Pressure in Five Minutes by Counting Your Breaths

For many of my patients, things like their blood pressure and pulse feel completely out of their control. They assume (and are, understandably, thankful) that their hearts keep beating without any involvement of their brains. They don't have to consciously think, "Beat, beat, beat . . ." Their hearts (and yours) do their jobs without being told.

This does not mean that you can't influence your heart rate or your blood pressure. You absolutely can influence both, and you can do it within a few minutes just by altering how you breathe.

Our heart rate is closely tied to our breathing rate. Normally, most of us breathe 14 to 16 times a minute, and our hearts beat about 60 times a minute. This breathing rate ensures that the cells in our bodies receive the oxygen they need and are able to discharge unneeded carbon dioxide. If our cells don't get enough oxygen, we breathe more quickly. If they do, we breathe more slowly. This all takes place without our awareness.

When we breathe slowly, our hearts beat slowly and we feel calmer. When we breathe quickly, our heart rate speeds up and we feel tense.

It's easy to prove this to yourself. Try it right now if you'd like. Take several quick, short breaths. How do you feel? Now breathe long, slowly and deeply. Now how do you feel? The first technique made you tense up, right? And the second one helped you calm down, right?

Long, slow, deep breathing is incredibly effective, not only for instilling a sense of calm, but also for dropping blood pressure. An Indian study of 23 patients with high blood pressure found that deep, slow breathing drops blood pressure within just five minutes![102] There are two branches of a nervous system that you rarely hear about but are crucial for controlling blood pressure.

Rachel's Journey to a Lasting Heart

Rachel was a challenge from the moment I first met her. She was referred by her internist because her blood pressure and cholesterol were high.

She was very well dressed. I learned that she was an attorney and quite well known in town. She enjoyed the reputation of battling fiercely in court and having "ice" in her veins. She slept only four hours a night, working on files and motions in the early morning. She had a personal trainer several times a week, and allotted him 30 minutes each meeting, as her schedule was regimented and full.

Several times during our first meeting she glanced at her watch, clearly wondering if she would make her next appointment. She even cut me off once or twice and finished my sentences.

I sent her for advanced labs and cardiac imaging that, fortunately, did not reveal any silent atherosclerosis. I told her she did not need to start medications just yet, but she really needed to concentrate on changing her lifestyle. I developed a plan for her that included a diet rich in whole, plant-based foods, at least six hours of sleep a night, and standing work breaks each hour. I mentioned the many benefits of a mind-body practice such as yoga. She scoffed, calling me "Swami Kahn." I was glad she had a sense of humor. That was a good sign.

When she returned for a blood pressure check, she surprised me. She told me that, initially, she had thought yoga would be about sitting in a lotus position on the floor and chanting. She didn't know that there were styles of yoga that were more athletic, and that yoga

These branches are called the parasympathetic nervous system (PNS) and the sympathetic nervous system (SNS). The PNS system is connected throughout the body by the vagus nerve. When it's activated, you feel relaxed and have a low heart rate and low blood pressure. The SNS is a web of the adrenal glands and nerve endings, and it has the opposite effect. Breathing slowly and deeply

combined movement and breath work to exercise both the body and the mind. We talked about yoga for a while, with her telling me what she found pleasing, and me giving pointers, such as pointing out the difference between a healthy slow burn class, suitable for beginners, and the hot Vinyasa practices that would be best for later on.

A month later she surprised me again. She had actually gone to one class a week for four weeks, finding that the teacher was her own age, a retired attorney, and a neighbor. She was struck by how much more relaxed the yoga teacher was, and how many fewer age lines and gray hairs were on the teacher's face and head. Now, in addition to yoga, she was also following a plant-based diet, too.

More startling, Rachel's systolic blood pressure (the top number) had fallen eight points. She asked if she could progress to a Vinyasa class, and I told her to go for it but to stick toward the back of the room and grab a spot near a wall for a break now and then.

During a visit two months later, Rachel was truly glowing. She was talking quickly and with enthusiasm about her poses, her teachers, studies she had tried, books she had read, and even her plans to go on a yoga beach retreat with her husband. On that visit her blood pressure was normal (<130/80) and it has remained normal since.

Rachel has also lost eight stubborn pounds and dropped a whole dress size. Colleagues often ask her what's new in her life. Although she avoided the need for blood pressure medicines, and I lost the need to see her in the clinic, I gained one very nice friend. She and her husband sometimes join my wife and I for dinner. What do we talk about? Yoga!

activates the PNS and turns off the SNS. The result is a lower heart rate, a lower blood pressure, and a more relaxed brain and heart.

Rx at a Glance

I understand what it's like to feel stressed. Every day I deal with deadlines, phone calls, pagers, and texts. Sometimes I wonder if my cell phone will ever stop ringing. Many of these calls are medical emergencies that I must respond to immediately. I cannot avoid the majority of these events, so I must find a way to cope, and breathing helps me to do that. If I feel my muscles start to knot up, I pause, take a breath in through my nose, let it out slowly through my mouth, and allow a moment of anxiety to pass. Try it!

To drop pressure, you want to slow your breathing so you are taking only six breaths a minute. To do so:

* **Close your eyes and bring your attention inward, toward your breath.**

* **Count in your head as you slowly inhale.**

* **Count in your head as you slowly exhale.**

* **Try to match your inhale to your exhale.** So if you inhale for a count of six, exhale for a count of six, too.

* **Going at your own pace and comfort level, try to slow your breathing so you are inhaling for a count of 10 and exhaling for a count of 10.** Make this your eventual goal, but don't stress yourself out over it. Remember: This is about instilling a state of calm. It's not a competition!

As you get used to this sequence, you can vary it. I usually do a 4-7-8 sequence: inhale through the nose for four seconds, hold for seven seconds, exhale through my mouth for eight. By breathing rhythmically in this way, you nudge your heart and the rest of your body to join you in the same rhythm. The technique shifts the autonomic nervous system away from the sympathetic predominance (which makes our hearts race and our palms sweaty when we face a stressful situation) and allows the parasympathetic nervous system to shine. Try it. It's a natural tranquilizer. Just three or four of these breaths and my heart rate slows, my nervous system calms, and I feel calm, cool, and collected. This is the easiest, most economical, and most effective stress reduction and mood-stabilizing program there is. And it only takes a minute! So 2-4-6-8, who do we appreciate?

Power Rx: Breathe through One Side of Your Nose

Many different styles of yoga teach a series of breathing exercises called "pranayama," or breath work.

One is alternate nostril breathing, where you breathe through one side of your nose at a time. At any given time, one side of our nose is dominant. If you close your eyes and pay attention to how the air flows in and out of your nose, you'll notice that you are primarily using either the right or the left nostril. It's probably not equal. And if you check again a few hours from now, you'll find that your dominant nostril has shifted. This is one of the natural rhythms of the body that takes place without our awareness. Scientists think we evolved with two nostrils (instead of one) because it improves our sense of smell. As you inhale, air rushes through your dominant nostril quickly, and through your non-dominant nostril slowly. The faster-traveling air communicates different smell information to the brain than the slower-traveling air.

Although there's little research to back it up, many believe that your dominant nostril stimulates more clarity in a corresponding area of the brain. So when you practice alternate nostril breathing, and you override the body's natural rhythms, you can stimulate different areas of the brain.

Indian scientists have been studying the effects of alternate nostril breathing almost as long as yogis have been practicing it, and they've come to some interesting findings. In one study, Indian researchers asked study subjects to do a series of yogic breath control exercises while their pulse rates were being monitored. The study participants did various types of alternate nostril breathing for 12 cycles. End result: Pulse rates slowed significantly, dropping an average of five pulses per minute.[103] A different study done on 15 patients with arrhythmia (abnormal heart rhythms) found that this type of breathing reduced ventricular repolarization dispersion, which is a pattern of disorganized heart electrical activity. The single nostril breathing brought order and coherence to the heart electricity, which is a goal for health and longevity.[104]

Rx at a Glance

There are many different ways to do alternate nostril breathing. If you've already learned one style and you enjoy it, keep it up. What follows is one simple technique:

* **Sit comfortably with your back straight.** Many people like to sit with their back against a wall for support.
* **Close the right nostril with your right thumb.**
* **Exhale through your left nostril.**
* **Inhale slowly through your left nostril.**
* **Close the left nostril with your thumb.**
* **Exhale through the right nostril.**
* **Inhale through the right nostril.**
* **Repeat back and forth for as many cycles as you wish.**

Power Rx: Breathe Out the Tension

Is there a way to calm down when you are in the middle of a stressful situation without anyone else noticing? Yes, there is. Again, a breathing technique comes to the rescue.

We are breathing all the time. No one around you knows whether you are paying attention to painful thoughts or to the natural in and out of your breathing. As a result, you can do most breathing exercises just about anywhere—even in the middle of a meeting at work—and, as long as you keep your eyes open, no one will be the wiser.

Rx at a Glance

The following technique is particularly helpful whenever you are experiencing some type of negativity, whether it be tension, anger, or something else:

* **Mentally gather up your negativity in the form of black smoke and breathe it right out your nose.**
* **Imagine that every inhale brings in white, radiant light that symbolizes peace, love, and joy.**
* **Imagine that both the black smoke and the white light come in and out of your nose, along with the air.** Or you can visualize them coming in and out of your heart. Try it both ways and see which you prefer.

It helps to do the technique several times in private before you try to do it when others are around. Familiarity breeds success, so practice it often, even when you are not particularly under stress.

Power Rx: Count Your Blessings

Not long ago, the University of California's Center for Greater Good launched a website called Thnx4.org that prompts users to take note of what they are thankful for, whether it be the actions of another person, a material possession, or a sunny day. When it unveiled the pilot version of the site, the Center for Greater Good asked users to complete surveys about how giving thanks affected their happiness, emotional resilience, and sense of life satisfaction. When the researchers there analyzed surveys taken before and after participants began making their gratitude entries, the upshot was clear: Taking the time to express their gratitude made them feel more thankful, and feeling more thankful also made them happier and more satisfied with life. Site users also reported a higher resilience to stress as well as fewer headaches, less congestion and stomach pain, and fewer sore throats.

This builds on past research that has found that counting one's blessings leads to health and happiness. When University of Connecticut psychologist Glen Affleck interviewed 287 people recovering from a heart attack, he found that people who found a positive benefit from their heart attack (such as learning an important life lesson from it or drawing closer to family as a result) fared better. They were less likely to suffer another heart attack within the next eight years.[105]

For more than a decade, University of California at Davis psychology professor Roger Emmons, PhD, has been studying how gratitude affects health and happiness. His research shows that a daily gratitude practice can:

* Boost immunity.
* Lower blood pressure.
* Encourage healthy behaviors like exercise and healthy eating.
* Improve sleep quality.[106]

And these results kick in within just a few weeks.

Rx at a Glance

Count your blessings at least once a day, using these pointers:

* **Use a journal, listing one or more things a day you feel thankful for.** Once a week, read over the journal. In lieu of a paper journal, consider using a site like Thnx4.org. If you don't want to write it down, at least do it in your head, and be intentional about it.

* **Ask yourself, "What am I grateful for today?** How have others helped me today? Who has been especially kind?"

* **Whenever possible, notice the exceptional people in your life rather than the exceptional things.** When users of Thnx4.org expressed thanks about other people, they were more likely to agree with the statement, "This made my whole day glorious." When they thought others had gone above and beyond the call of duty, they felt even happier.

* **Make a habit of noticing the small acts of kindness unfolding all around you.** When a stranger smiles and tells you to have a great day, think, "Kind!" Do the same with that motorist who graciously allows you to merge into traffic, as well as the friend who called just to check up on you.

Power Rx: Meditate Your Stress Away

Meditation is nothing more than focusing your mind on a single point to enhance awareness and mindfulness.

You can focus it on your breath, on a mantra (such as "om," "I have enough," "aha"), on the sensations of your body, or on a concept such as love, patience, or equanimity.

The idea is that, once you focus on your breathing or something else, you are not focusing on all of the things that tend to cause you stress. As a result, your mind automatically calms down and a sense of peace automatically arises. If you meditate on love, you'll also feel a sense of warmth at your heart.

There are several methods of teaching meditation. Transcendental meditation (TM) was made famous by the Beatles and is the most well known and researched of the practices, particularly at the Maharishi University in Iowa. The TM technique involves meditating on a mantra for 20 minutes twice a day while seated comfortably with the eyes shut. Does it work in heart patients? Does it ever! One study done at the Medical College of Wisconsin found that people who practiced TM regularly were 48 percent less likely to have a heart attack or stroke than others who took health education classes instead. Blood pressure dropped by five mmHg in the TM group, and their anger also lessened significantly.[107] A medication that dropped heart attack rates 48 percent would sell billions of dollars a year, but sadly only medication, and not meditation, is recommended to most heart patients.

The results were so dramatic that lead researcher Robert Schneider, MD, commented that meditation "is a technique that turns on the body's own pharmacy—to repair and maintain itself."

Rx at a Glance

There are as many styles of meditation as there are of yoga. I recommend you try several to see which one feels the most comfortable for you. In addition to TM, another popular form of meditation called "mindfulness" has also garnered a lot of research. As a result, Jon Kabat Zinn's Mindfulness Based Stress Reduction (MBSR) program, originally pioneered at the University of Massachusetts, is now offered at hospitals around the country and is often covered by insurance. You also might find classes taught locally at yoga studios or meditation centers. A number of apps and online videos are available, too. The Isha Foundation, in particular, has made meditation training available online by various video teaching courses that can be accessed for free at www.ishafoundation.org.

No matter which style you try, use these pointers:

* **Start with what you can handle.** Don't make perfect the enemy of good. Rather than continually putting off meditation because you don't have a spare 20 minutes, just sit down, close your eyes, and focus single-pointedly on something for whatever amount of time you have. Even just a few minutes can help immensely.

* **Don't become self-critical.** Meditation is a form of concentration. It takes practice to get better at it. Congratulate yourself every single time you catch your mind wandering off. Gently bring it back with a smile. Each time you try to meditate, it's like training a muscle. The effort you put into one session will pay off the next time you sit down to meditate.

Power Rx: Meditate Your Anger Away, Too

We know that anger activates the fight-or-flight response, quickly marshaling those dangerous stress hormones into the bloodstream. It speeds up the heart rate and gives us a burst of energy, but it comes at a cost. Anger speeds up the formation of plaque in the arteries and spikes blood pressure.

Good thing there's an antidote, one that is easier to cultivate than you might think: love.

Researchers from the University of North Carolina at Chapel Hill and the University of California divided 65 people into two groups. One group learned a form of meditation called "loving kindness." The other group was placed on a waiting list for meditation training.

Before, during, and after the training, researchers measured study participants' heart rates and breathing patterns. They also measured vagal tone—which is a measure of the parasympathetic nervous system (the calming one), and a sign of relaxation and health. Not only did the meditators report increases in awe, gratitude, and amusement, they also said they felt more socially connected to others and more in tune with the people around them.

End result: improvements in vagal tone and a calmer nervous system.[108]

Rx at a Glance

Loving kindness is a great meditation to do every day. It will transform your relationships with others. Perhaps you will do it every morning before you start your day. Or you might do it at night before bed. Here's what you do:

* **Sit quietly, close your eyes, and bring your attention inward.**

* **To calm your mind, spend a few moments focusing on your breathing, following the breath in and out.**

* **Bring one person to mind, preferably someone you find exceptionally easy to love.** Imagine this person in front of you and cultivate a warm, light, loving feeling in your heart.

* **Think about how you and this person want the same out of life.** You both want to be happy. You both want to avoid suffering.

* **As you exhale, imagine that the peace travels from your heart to theirs in the form of white light.** Believe that this light contains healing energy and that it has the power to bring this person happiness.

* **Spend a few moments visualizing this, feeling a deep sense of joy** over the idea of giving happiness and peace to someone else.

* **Then continue to do the meditation, bringing another person to mind, then another and another.**

Power Rx: Cuddle with a Pet

When many of my patients told me about the special bonds they had with their pets, I wondered: Could pets help prevent heart disease? I went to the National Library of Medicine and soon found my answer: Yes! Many years ago, Dr. Erika Friedman studied 92 patients who had been admitted to a cardiac care unit for a heart attack or a serious angina heart pain episode. She gathered information on pet ownership. A year after their discharge from the cardiac unit, 94 percent of the pet owners were still alive, whereas only 71 percent of the patients without pets were.[111]

Other research shows that merely talking to or petting a dog can help drive down blood pressure, a phenomenon known as "the pet effect." This effect holds even if the dog isn't yours—and, amazingly, even if you don't like dogs.[112] People are better able to complete a stressful task if they have a pet with them, and they find their pets more emotionally soothing than friends or family.[113]

Indeed, pets also seem to have an amazing impact on stress, cholesterol levels, and blood pressure. Part of the effect probably comes from their unconditional love. Pets are always happy to see you, forgive you when you are not your best self, and seem to listen to you no matter what you have to say. Part of it perhaps stems from their loyalty, playful attention, and unconditional love, and part may even come from their energy field. As I explained in Part One, our heart is powered with an electrical current that creates a field of energy about us that can be measured up to several feet away. In fact, we can interact with the energy fields of other living creatures, such as our pets, within this radius. Pets generally have a calmer energy field than we do, which might calm our energy fields, thus stabilizing our heart rhythms.

Rx at a Glance

Of course, this advice will only work for you if you happen to love dogs or other types of pets. If you do:

* **Consider adopting your pet from a shelter.** This can save you hundreds of dollars, and it also allows you to come home with an older pet that is already house trained and much less destructive than a puppy.

* **Volunteer with therapy dogs or an animal shelter.** This allows you to couple the benefits of associating with dogs with the benefits of volunteering—and without the responsibility and expense of ownership!

Power Rx: Get Busy

Sexual intimacy and activity can be both preventive and healing in heart disease. Men who have sex at least twice a week reduce their risk of heart attack by half, compared to men who have sex only about once a month. Not even aspirin has that kind of effect.[114] Similar studies are not available in women, but there's no reason to assume sex isn't just as good for the fairer sex.

Rx at a Glance

Many people with heart issues want to have sex, but they worry about dropping dead of a heart attack while in the process. Since you might have the same concerns, I thought I'd reassure you with some advice and guidelines:

* **Sexual intimacy is about as taxing on the body as light exercise that gets your heart rate to 130 beats per minute.** If you feel safe while power walking or climbing two flights of stairs, then you should feel just as safe in the bedroom.

* **In clinically stable individuals, the risk of heart attacks and death during sex is very low.**

* **If you are worried, ask for a treadmill or bicycle stress test.** If you can complete a stress test without any issues, you can also have sex without any issues.

* **Heart disease narrows the arteries all over your body, including the ones to your genitals.** As a result, many men with heart disease also experience erectile dysfunction. If you are on nitroglycerin, then medicines used to treat erectile dysfunction are not recommended. Usually, however, alternatives can be found. For instance, testosterone replacement therapy is one possible alternative that can be used in place of erectile dysfunction medications.

Power Rx: Sleep Seven to Eight Hours at Night

Every day our bodies are challenged by stress, toxins, radiation, variable nutrition and hydration, and other factors that can deplete our ability to perform optimally. To prevent cumulative wear and tear, we need to sleep so that our bodies can produce antioxidants, heal wounds, repair DNA, and encourage the activity of an anti-aging enzyme called telomerase. Also, during sleep, our levels of stress hormones such as cortisol and adrenaline drop.

How important is sleep duration? In a study of over 80,000 women in the Women's Health Initiative, women with both insomnia and prolonged sleep had the highest rate of heart disease, while the midrange sleepers, those at the sweet spot of seven to eight hours, had the lowest rates, almost one-half lower.[115]

One disorder of sleep that is of particular concern is obstructive sleep apnea. Sleep apnea is linked to hypertension, heart failure, stroke, and lung disease, and may double the risk of heart disease and heart deaths if untreated. Markers of inflammation are increased, too. Because overweight people are more likely to develop sleep apnea (though thin folks can have it, too), it is increasing in frequency. Hallmarks of sleep apnea include snoring, excessive daytime fatigue, and interruptions in breathing during sleep. If you think you might have sleep apnea, seek out a trained specialist in sleep medicine and get tested and treated.

Rx at a Glance

Perhaps the hardest aspect of good health is achieving at least seven (but preferably eight) hours of uninterrupted sleep at night. Poor sleep may have many causes: sleep apnea, untreated depression or anxiety, late night eating and computer and TV stimulation, a bedroom that isn't sufficiently dark, pets that jump on or off the bed or curl up on your head, small children, or, of course, a noisy phone that beeps every time a text comes in from someone still awake in another time zone. The health benefits of adequate sleep on mental function, weight control, and overall wellness are great.

Sleep is important, and can greatly benefit your mental function, weight control, heart health, and overall wellness. Don't take sleep problems lightly. Use these tips to rest well:

* **If you think you might have sleep apnea, see your health care provider as soon as possible.** Chances are, your health care provider will prescribe a sleep study that you can actually do at home. You just attach a little device to yourself as you sleep. If you test positive for sleep apnea, your health care provider will probably prescribe a device called a CPAP (Continuous Positive Airway Pressure) to wear at night. This is a mask that you wear. It blows air into the nose and/or mouth, keeping airways open.

* **Avoid electromagnetic frequency around bedtime.** Our thoughts and other brain activity all arise from the bioelectrical activity of neurons, and the electromagnetic waves emitted from cell phones and laptop computers using wireless frequencies can change our brain waves, turning down the delta waves we need for stage two sleep, an effect that may last as long as an hour after you've turned off your phone.[116] This will help to prevent tossing and turning.

* **Dark and cool bedrooms may help induce better sleep.**

* **Don't watch TV or use computers for at least a half hour before bed.** The stimulation can keep your mind awake, and the light emitted from these devices also tricks your brain into thinking it's daytime.

* **Stop eating two to three hours before bedtime.**

* **Try herbal therapies.** Take one of the following about 30 minutes before bed: melatonin (1 to 5 mg),

valerian root (150 to 600 mg in escalating doses), L-theanine (200 to 400 mg), or magnesium (250 to 500 mg, preferably of the chelated forms) if you have insomnia.

Power Rx: Walk in the Sun for 15 Minutes

You already know that walking is good for your heart. You also know that vitamin D, produced in your skin when it interacts with sunlight, is good for the heart.

Here's one more reason to walk in the sun: blood pressure. When our skin is exposed to sunlight, a compound is released in the blood that helps to lower blood pressure. This substance, nitric oxide, is the same substance that makes an arugula salad so good for you. Researchers at the University of Edinburgh studied the blood pressure of 24 volunteers as they sat under ultraviolet light for 20 minutes. Blood pressure dropped for an entire hour following exposure to UV light, but not when men tanned using lamps that didn't emit UV.[117] While I am not recommending you frequent tanning centers or purchase a tanning bed, the role of sunshine on blood pressure and artery health is backed by science. Sunlight might also help lift depression by activating the pineal gland and the body's natural circadian rhythms. Walking outdoors helps you get to know your neighbors, which helps to reverse social isolation. Sunshine and fresh air, especially combined with the physical activity of walking, can heal your body and soul.

Rx at a Glance

* **Make a habit of walking outdoors once a day.**
* **Go barefoot.** If you can walk barefoot in the grass or on the Earth (a practice called grounding, which you'll learn more about on page 215), you may also lower inflammation.

* **Stroll after meals.** If you walk after a meal, you'll blunt the rise of post-meal blood sugar levels, reducing your risk for developing diabetes.

* **Immerse yourself in nature.** You might find certain environments more calming than others, especially walking trails through wooded areas or along bodies of water.

Power Rx: Embrace Volunteer Work

When we help others, we receive something in return: a mood boost and a sense of connection and purpose. That translates to less stress and better health. Researchers have found that people who volunteer their time to help others:

* **Have lower blood pressure.** Research out of Carnegie Mellon University finds that older adults who volunteer 200 or more hours a year reduce their risk of developing high blood pressure by 40 percent.[118]

* **Feel less pain.** When patients with chronic pain help others, their pain diminishes.[119]

* **Live longer.** Older adults who volunteer live an average of two years longer than their peers who don't.[120]

Plus volunteer work makes the world a better place. There has probably been a time in your life when you've benefitted from the kindness of others. Maybe a teacher took extra time with you, or perhaps a plumber friend fixed your toilet for free. Think of how fortunate you are to have received so much kindness from others. Now it's time to pay it forward.

Ask the Holistic Heart Doc:

I've been told to get up earlier in the morning in order to fit in exercise. Now you're telling me to get enough sleep. How do I accomplish both?

This is a tough choice, one I find myself making every day. What to do? Sleep more? Or exercise more? I debate in my head whether I should wake 60 to 90 minutes early to grab a gym bag and head for the health club, wake up 45 to 60 minutes early to work out at home, or grab every last bit of sleep to reach seven to eight hours of rest.

What do I do? A little bit of each. If I'm well rested and I was able to get to bed at a reasonable time, then I'm up early and at the gym for the 5:00 a.m. fitness class. On the other hand, if I find myself at the hospital late into the night helping a patient in distress, I might choose to get up only 15 minutes early and do a quick Tabata routine (page 173) before work. Also, if I get up for the 5 a.m. fitness class on one day, I'll usually reward myself the following morning by sleeping in.

Rx at a Glance

To reap the benefits of volunteering:

* **Start with any amount of time.** Even just five minutes once a week is better than none. Start with whatever you can fit in.
* **Think small.** Every day, set out to make someone else's day a little better.
* **Think about giving.** Just thinking about it, research shows, makes you more likely to do it.[121]

Power Rx: Take Vitamin Y (Try Yoga)

In Chapter 8, I told you about the wonderful physical fitness benefits of yoga. Here I'm talking mainly about the mental ones.

Yoga is much more than a series of postures that stretch, strengthen, and align the body. It's really an entire lifestyle, one that is defined by union: Of the mind and body, of motion and breath, of each of us to the other.

The practice originated in India but has grown rapidly across the Western world. Now, no matter where you live, you probably have access to classes at a yoga studio, a fitness center, or even a house of worship. A friend who teaches yoga told me that her father's church just added yoga classes. She could not get him to join her yoga studio, but he signed up at church. I told her it was a victory for wellness. Many online and DVD training materials are also available. I even have several yoga training applications on my smartphone.

There are several ways yoga brings about a sense of calm:

Body awareness. As you move through each pose you are encouraged to focus on your body—on pulling your hip one way and anchoring your foot another. By focusing your mind on your alignment, you automatically stop focusing on your to-do list or ruminating on all of the irritations in your life.

Breath work. Many yoga classes teach breathing exercises called pranayama that help to still the mind and instill a sense of euphoria.

Chanting. Similar to breath work, the chanting done in some classes can help to activate the vagus nerve that runs from your heart to your brain, instilling a deep sense of calm.

Meditation and relaxation. Some classes also teach you to meditate on your breath, on a mantra, or on love. No matter the object of your meditation, this can bring a sense of peace.

Researchers have studied yoga for many years, finding that a regular practice increases the output of the parasympathetic nervous system (the nervous system that brings you calm and peace) and decreases activity of the sympathetic nervous system (the one where the trigger for your fight-or-flight response resides). This leads to improvement in a measure of heart function called heart rate variability, which is measured by the time between heartbeats on breathing in and out. It is healthier to have your heart rate swing up and down quite a bit as you breathe. That means healthy nerves are supplying the heart and arteries. Improvements in heart rate variability occurring with yoga are suspected to improve longevity.

Yoga has also been shown to:

* Improve blood sugar control by increasing insulin release from the pancreas.
* Lower cholesterol and triglyceride levels.
* Assist in weight loss.
* Lower blood pressure.
* Improve lung function.
* Decrease asthma attacks and reduce the need for asthma medication.
* Reduce the need for blood pressure, cholesterol, and blood sugar–lowering medications.

One study even found that yoga brought about improvements of coronary blockages.[122] Recent elegant research on gene expression has shown that a regular yoga practice modifies gene output in white blood cells and may boost immune health.[123] There has even been research indicating that the blood of yoga practitioners contains a higher level of antioxidants and lower levels of markers of oxidative stress.[124]

Rx at a Glance

Yoga is so good for you that I like to call it vitamin Y. I recommend you take it regularly. I practice yoga several times a week and enjoy the hot room, the pulsating music, the detoxifying sweat, and the moments of meditative calm and rest at the end (savasana, or Corpse Pose). I have recently added Kundalini yoga and the energy renewal that this seems to provide is welcome.

There are many styles of yoga. Try a few and see which you like the most. Here's a description of some of the more popular ones, along with their specific benefits:

* **Restorative and Yin yoga.** In these forms, postures are held for a long time and props are often used to help you relax. These classes are very slow moving, and are ideal if you have injuries, aches and pains, or overall body tightness. They are also a wonderful way to unwind after a stressful day.

* **Kundalini yoga.** Relatively new in the West, this style combines some movement, chanting, meditation, breath work, and even gongs to provide a physical and spiritual energy overhaul that can be invigorating.

* **Hatha yoga.** This is probably the most common form of yoga. It includes a well-rounded balance of asanas (yoga postures), breathing exercises, and purification techniques such as meditation, sweating, and nasal washing. Some Hatha classes carry the name of the yoga master or yoga ashram that brought them to the West. For instance, rather than Hatha, your teacher might say the style is Iyengar or Kripalu style. Iyengar-style yoga uses lots of props, and it's great for people with aches, pains, and body limitations.

* **Hot yoga.** If you are into fitness, hot yoga might be for you. This style of yoga combines two things that are exceptionally good for your heart health: heat (these styles are taught in a room often more than 100°F) and movement. Despite popular belief, extreme heat

is very good for the heart. Check out the Power Rx on page 212 for more. After a hot yoga class, you'll feel stretched, strengthened, and cleansed.

Power Rx: Try Tai Chi

Tai chi is a gentle, meditative exercise with origins in Chinese martial arts. It involves flowing arm movements, breathing, balance, shifting of weight, and focused awareness.

The movements are gentle, making it especially suitable for the elderly and heart disease patients. Like yoga, it definitely can get you fit and improve your balance and range of motion, but it's main heart benefits are emotional. It will calm and center you, allowing you to leave class with a smile on your face.

When researchers from Tufts Medical Center in Boston analyzed the existing research on tai chi—which included a total of 40 studies done on thousands of participants—they concluded that tai chi significantly reduced stress, anxiety, and depression.[125]

Rx at a Glance

Sure, there are books, videos, and online tutorials, but the best (and least stressful!) way to learn tai chi is a class. If you are intrigued, check to see if there is a health center near you where tai chi is taught. You'll likely find classes at the following places:

* Hospital wellness centers.
* Martial arts studios.
* Yoga studios.

Power Rx: Get a Little Breathing Help from Your Apps

One of the benefits of technology has been this: It allows many more people to access the benefits of breathing, relaxation, and meditation exercises. If you don't have classes near you, don't have time to get to a class, or just don't feel comfortable taking a class, then Meditation 2.0 is for you.

A number of new apps and gadgets are now on the market. I've recommended a few to my patients, and they rave about them. They're great for people who love technology and who also prefer to do meditation and breathing exercises in the privacy of their homes.

Rx at a Glance

There are many, many devices and apps, but there are two in particular that I recommend:

* **RESPeRATE.** This is an FDA-approved device for blood pressure control that focuses on rhythmic breathing and mind relaxation. You wear a portable computerized device. Its chest sensors pick up on your breathing pattern. Then an earpiece plays a melody designed to help you naturally change your breathing pattern for the better. You almost can't help but synchronize your breathing to the tones played by the device. I have recommended this device with success to patients. It costs around $300, but it might save you about that much or more in medication. Many of my patients were able to reduce the dosage of or stop taking some medicines altogether after using this device. You can learn more at www.resperate.com.

* **HeartMath.** This is a software package you load on your smartphone or computer. It includes guided exercises of breathing and concentration that help you achieve coherence of the mind and heart. It has been shown to lower stress hormone levels and improve heart rate variability. You can learn more at www.heartmathstore.com. Prices range from $99 to $189.

Power Rx: Join a Group of Like-Minded People

We're social creatures and appear to thrive when we have strong bonds. For example, in research involving more than 300,000 people, the stronger an individual's social network, the less likely that person was to die prematurely. In fact, survival in the most socially connected individuals was improved by 50 percent compared to those without strong social ties.[126] In other words: Friendship is a powerful healing force.

The power of small groups is best told as a story about a huge church in Los Angeles. The Saddleback Church is an enormous congregation with more than 30,000 members. It's actually much more than one church. There are really several campuses and locations, all headed by Pastor Rick Warren.

Until recently, many Saddleback events centered around ice cream socials, hot dog parties, and doughnuts. After the congregants and Pastor Rick ballooned up in size, Pastor Rick decided to do something about it. He gathered a panel of doctors, including Mark Hyman, MD, Daniel Amen, MD, and Mehmet Oz, MD, and asked for their help in converting the church's 5,000 or so Bible groups into vehicles for better health. The result: the Daniel Plan.

In the first week, 16,000 members of the church signed up. They received lectures, videos, handouts, and activities geared to movement and healthy lifestyles.

While some of the plan involves healthy eating and exercise, the main power of the program has to do with the bonding that occurs when people with similar goals meet in small groups. Loneliness is a stressor on the heart, much as depression is. When you join a group of like-minded people, you feel a sense of oneness, and you also have a community of people who are there to encourage you to meet your goal.

For the Daniel Plan, the core activity was using the small Bible study groups as discussion points. Members often went shopping, eating, and walking together. In one year, they collectively lost more than 250,000 pounds. Plus, everything from blood pressure to blood cholesterol improved.

I had the pleasure of bringing the Daniel Plan to my synagogue, the first Jewish congregation to use the structure and adapt the theology to our faith. The message of healthy, clean eating, movement, sleep, and stress management really resonated with our community. The Daniel Plan now includes several of my articles on its website, which is a great honor.

Rx at a Glance

You don't have to participate in the Daniel Plan to benefit from the power of small groups. Anything that connects you to others will help. Use this advice:

* **Get to know your neighbors.** The impersonal nature of modern neighborhoods, virtual workplaces, and online communication has separated us to some degree from close bonds with others. The more connected you feel to others who live near you, the more you'll be able to lean on them in times of need.

* **Join a group that you believe in.** It might be a service organization such as Kiwanis or Lions Club or an exercise group that is raising money for a cause.

* **Bring the Daniel Plan or another healthy initiative to your place of worship.** Set up a wellness committee and review the Daniel Plan website. Consider guidelines for healthy foods at meetings, walking clubs, and stress-reducing breaks. Bring in a speaker from a fitness club, the American Heart Association, or a wellness center.

There is an African proverb that states, "If you want to walk fast, walk alone. If you want to walk far, walk together." Grabbing someone's hand and walking together through challenges may be the most powerful health tool of all.

Power Rx: Try Waon Therapy

We have all seen the warning signs posted by most saunas advising caution for heart patients. These are usually steam saunas kept at high temperatures. Research scientists in both Finland and Japan have questioned this advice, however, and have performed and published many studies, specifically looking at how heat affects heart patients. Generally, dry saunas have been used and the temperature has been kept to 60°C or 140°F maximum.

The most data is from Japan, where they have used a special kind of dry sauna known as infrared sauna. This sauna penetrates the skin with deeper energy than standard dry saunas. For more than 20 years, doctors in Japan have been testing the benefits of infrared dry sauna therapy in some of the sickest heart and vascular patients, and they've published nearly 20 research articles showing this is a major breakthrough.

They've used a technique called waon therapy (pronounced WOW-n), from the Japanese words *wa* for soothing and *on* for warmth, or so-called soothing warmth therapy. The way it works: Patients sit in an infrared sauna set at 60°C (140°F) for 15 minutes, followed by resting outside the sauna for 30 minutes, wrapped in towels. People are encouraged to drink water to compensate for the perspiration.

As I've mentioned, the lining of your arteries is a single layer of cells called your endothelium. Acting as much more than a simple barrier for blood cells, these cells produce dozens of compounds that cause arteries to resist developing plaque, blood clots, or constriction. Waon therapy has been shown to improve the function of these cells and the blood flow they carry.

In an amazing study of 129 patients with bad heart problems, patients treated with waon therapy at least two times a week were compared to similar patients who did not get the soothing warmth therapy. Over five years of follow-up, the rate of re-hospitalization and death was half in the waon-treated patients compared to the others![127, 128] As you know, if a drug reduced hospitalization and death by 50 percent, it would easily be a billion-dollar winner.

If waon therapy is so beneficial in heart patients, why haven't you heard of it? And why isn't it used more? In my opinion, it's partly due to the fact that many health care providers aren't familiar with the strong data supporting it, and partly due to the fact that low-tech treatments such as this one get buried by expensive and glitzy therapies that may not prove to be as beneficial.

Rx at a Glance

This therapy is probably easier for you to access than you might think.

* **Consult your health insurance carrier.** Waon therapy might be covered. Or if you have a Health Savings Account, you can use that to cover the cost of sessions.

* **Aim for the same length of a session found to be effective in the research:** 15 minutes in the infrared sauna followed by 30 minutes resting while wrapped in towels.

* **Consider buying your own unit.** A home infrared sauna unit can be purchased for around $750 to

$5,000, depending on whether it is portable or permanent and on how many people it is designed to seat. I have one in my home and it has become one of the most relaxing family rituals.

* **See if you can rent time at an infrared sauna.** There are wellness centers where I live that rent a waon therapy spot for about $20 for half an hour.

If you can't get to an infrared sauna, try the traditional dry sauna at your typical gym. You can probably get many of the same benefits.

Power Rx: Try Acupuncture

Acupuncture is a key component of traditional Chinese medicine that is now widely available in North America. It has been used in many treatments of heart disease, and many studies support its use.

It involves penetrating the skin with needles that are then manipulated by manual or electrical means. It's based on the idea that there is an energy, or qi, that flows through the body. Blockages in this flow can cause disease, and acupuncture helps correct these imbalances.

The use of acupuncture has been supported by the National Institutes of Health, the National Center for Complementary and Alternative Medicine, and the World Health Organization.

The National Library of Medicine lists over 19,000 studies on acupuncture, with more than 500 focused on cardiovascular conditions. Acupuncture has been studied as a therapy for angina pectoris, an uncomfortable chest discomfort that develops when inadequate blood flow reaches the heart muscles. This is usually caused by narrowed heart arteries. When researchers analyzed more than 16 studies, they found that acupuncture plus medication worked better than conventional drugs alone at preventing heart attacks and reducing the frequency and duration of angina symptoms.[129]

Acupuncture may also help drop blood pressure by increasing the action of the calming parasympathetic nervous system and decreasing the action of the stress-inducing sympathetic nervous system.

Rx at a Glance

If you're interested in giving acupuncture a try:

* **Sign up for the long term.** Acupuncture seems to only work as you are getting it. Subsequent studies have shown some benefit goes away when acupuncture is stopped.

* **Ask friends and relatives for referrals.** The American Association of Acupuncture and Chinese Medicine is also a good resource to find licensed acupuncturists (www.aaaomonline.org).

* **Give the treatments time.** You should notice an improvement in blood pressure, chest pain, and/or stress levels within three to four treatments.

* **Check if your insurance covers your treatments.** If it doesn't, you can save money by visiting a community acupuncturist. These practitioners work publicly, with all of their patients in the same room. This means you will have little privacy, but you'll also have a smaller bill to pay at checkout.

Power Rx: Ground Yourself

The Earth emits negatively charged electrons, and an increasingly popular treatment called "Earthing" (also sometimes called "grounding") is based on the idea that the Earth's negative charge is a stabilizing force for good health. This all sounds pretty far-out, and I was skeptical at first. There is not nearly as much evidence proving benefits of this therapy as there is for acupuncture and many other prescriptions in this book. Still, after reading all the published scientific studies on this topic, I began incorporating more Earthing strategies into my life. Should you do the same? That's up to you. Here's what you need to know.

Earthing refers to the attempt to increase our contact with the Earth's surface by walking barefoot outside, sleeping in contact with the Earth, and generally being connected to the Earth's conductive system as often as possible. According to Dr. James Oschman, one of the biggest proponents of Earthing, the Earth supplies us with a constant source of electrons, the most powerful antioxidants around.[130] To soak them in, all we need to do is connect with the planet, skin to Earth, so to speak.

Preliminary research suggests that grounding might have anti-inflammatory effects, soothe pain, improve sleep and heart rate variability, and calm the nervous system.[131] One recent small study assessed the effects of grounding on blood thickening, also known as viscosity. When many heart attacks, strokes, and blood clots occur, it is due to the blood thickening too much and forming dangerous blood clots. The grounding reduced viscosity in ten study participants.[132]

Rx at a Glance

The jury is still out on whether Earthing offers a strong heart benefit, but it can't hurt. Plus, most of the activities that increase your contact with the Earth are naturally calming and enjoyable. For instance:

* **Walk barefoot, on grass, sand, or soil, whenever possible.** In addition to grounding yourself, you'll be stimulating your feet, which, in and of itself, is very relaxing.

* **Relax on the ground.** Make snow angels with your kids. Rest in the grass or sit by the shade of a tree.

* **Move the earth.** Many people love to garden, and it's a great stress reliever.

* **Consider purchasing grounding sheets.** These are bedsheets that are laced with a fine conductive wire lattice that is wired into a plug attached to a grounded outlet. These grounding or Earthing sheets connect the outside Earth to your bed if the plug is indeed grounded, which is easy to check. Is the outlet three pronged? Then you're grounded, and the sheets are working their magic.

YOUR FINAL EMOTIONAL HEALTH RX

You just read several lifestyle suggestions, most of which cost zero dollars. Many of them you can do at home, right now. And they are amazingly effective. I can't emphasize the importance of stress relief for heart health strongly enough.

Which prescriptions you decide to incorporate into your life will depend a lot on your personality, lifestyle, and current state of emotional health. If you describe yourself as a high-stress, type A person, the breathing exercises should become one of your main practices. If you are the type of person who embraces everything from the mind-body field, then acupuncture and Earthing are probably for you. Just try these strategies with an open mind. Some will stick. Others won't. That's okay. What's most important is that you find a few strategies that help you feel calmer, happier, and more at peace.

Remember Dr. Friedman? I mentioned him at the beginning of this chapter. He's the doctor who coined the term "type A." And he was type A himself. Even as he was researching the connection between stress and heart disease, he was suffering the effects of his own stress. In the mid-1950s, he suffered his first of two heart attacks at age 45. Those heart attacks were a wake-up call. Along with his research findings, they encouraged him to take steps to reduce his stress. You know what? The stress reduction worked. Friedman went on to live over 40 more years, dying in 2001 at the age of 91. You can do the same.

Chapter 10

Your Eco Rx

When most people hear the word "toxic," they think of sludge that runs off a chemical plant, the stuff that coats the ground of a garbage site, or neighborhoods like Love Canal near Niagara Falls, New York, where residents were poisoned by contaminated groundwater.

Most don't think about products found at the average grocery store and especially not common objects found at home, perhaps a home much like yours, and that the toxins in these products can harm their hearts.

Let's take a walk through your home and see.

First, open your refrigerator. Look inside. Do you see any plastic water bottles, perhaps ones you grab on your way to the gym? Now, walk over to your stove. What kind of a frying pan do you use? Does it have a nonstick coating?

Now walk to the bathroom. Look around. Is there any makeup? Body lotion? Toothpaste? A bottle of air freshener?

Let's go from there to the living room. Have you purchased any new furniture lately, perhaps something made with particleboard?

If your home is like most—including my own until recently—

the answers to the questions I just posed are probably, "Yes, yes, yes, yes, yes, yes, and yes."

Perhaps much like you, not long ago I was drinking water from plastic bottles that had been sitting in the sun for days, drinking hot coffee from Styrofoam cups, microwaving snacks in plastic containers, and washing my hair with shampoos that had more chemical names than my hospital pharmacy. However, when I became a student of the medical aspects of the relationship between our home environment and our health, I started to make changes.

More than 80,000 chemicals are used to make common products we all use daily when cooking, cleaning, and caring for our own bodies. Most did not exist 100 years ago. Only 1,000 have been studied for their effects on human health, and many of them have already been shown to be dangerous.

These chemicals leak into the air inside your home in the form of fumes, migrate into your food and beverages, and seep into your skin. As a result, researchers have found more than 200 chemicals in breast milk and in umbilical cord blood. They've also discovered them in the bloodstreams of newborn infants, children, teens, and adults. Some of these chemicals, like DDT, were banned years ago, but they are still showing up in our blood and they still contaminate the water and soil. Some of them contribute to health problems like low fertility or thyroid dysfunction, which indirectly affect our hearts for the worse. Others directly contribute to heart disease by turning up inflammation, raising blood pressure, or hardening the arteries.

But you're not helpless. You can do something about it.

Power Rx: Open Your Windows to Reduce Indoor Air Pollution

The air inside your home might be even more polluted than the air in some of the world's dirtiest cities.

That's no exaggeration.

We spend up to 90 percent of our time indoors, which means much of the 3,000 to 6,000 gallons of air we inhale daily comes from air in our homes or places of employment (which may be just as polluted).

Where does all of this indoor air pollution come from? Some of it seeps in from the outdoors and then gets locked inside, where it builds up over time. This may be especially true if you live in a newer home with tight seals and state-of-the-art windows that don't allow air to escape.

But a lot of it is created inside our homes. Consider the following sources of indoor air pollution:

* New furniture, carpeting, and mattresses are created with dozens of different chemicals, including formaldehyde, a carcinogen. Think about the smell of new carpeting or of a new mattress. That smell comes from chemical fumes that are escaping from the new piece of furniture.

* Chloroform, a carcinogenic fume that escapes from bleach bottles and other cleaning products, runs rampant in our homes. Air samples taken from various homes reveal that indoor air has, on average, 10 times more concentrated chloroform than outdoor air.

* The floral scent from any air freshener you might spray to mask an odor comes from a chemical compound called phthalates known to disrupt the endocrine system (more on phthalates on page 229). Of 14 brands of air fresheners tested by the National Resources Defense Council, all but two had high levels of phthalates. This spray may also contain volatile organic compounds—the same compounds that are a component of smog—as well as the carcinogens benzene and formaldehyde.

And there are dozens of other possible sources ranging from hair spray to candles to fumes that come off the nonstick coating on your cookware. While any one of these chemicals might be considered harmless in small amounts, the caustic brew they create when mixed together, concentrated, and left to build up in an airtight home creates a potent recipe for heart disease, a team of researchers found a few years ago. To study the health effects of indoor air, these scientists from Denmark and Sweden did an interesting experiment. For two days, the researchers measured certain markers of health in 21 healthy, elderly couples while the couples performed their normal routines at home. Then for two more days, the researchers continued to measure the same markers of health, but this time they filtered the air inside the couples' homes.

The results were startling. The air filters were able to remove up to 9,000 particles per cubic centimeter from the air in each couple's home, resulting in a near immediate eight percent improvement in the functioning of the small blood vessels.[133] This improvement may be enough to lower blood pressure, reduce angina pain, or improve blood flow.

Why? It goes back to those endothelial cells that line the walls of the blood vessels. These cells control blood flow, reduce clotting, keep arteries clear, reduce swelling, and even form new blood vessels. When we inhale tiny air pollution particles, however, these bits of debris make their way into the bloodstream, damaging these important cells.

Rx at a Glance

If you suffer from chronic headaches, dry eyes, fatigue, allergies, or asthma, chances are there are toxins lurking inside your home, and the fix is quite simple. Open your windows, start a fan, and circulate that air. Doing so can quickly drop the level of indoor air pollution, not only helping you feel better, but also protecting your heart. This is especially important to do when you're cleaning or

Mary's Journey to a Lasting Heart

Mary, a friend of my parents, was in her early 70s when she first came to see me as a patient. At first she merely wanted to know whether her blood pressure and cholesterol levels were in the healthy range, but I was struck by the number of allergies she'd listed on her intake form: all perfumes, all fragrant detergents, all scented clothes softeners, metals, tape, latex.

When I asked her about the long and unusual list, she told me that she organized her life so she could avoid interacting with large crowds where she would likely interact with some of the offending agents she reacted to. Her friends knew that a night out with Mary meant no cologne or perfume, and that even then, odds were that something might happen to trigger wheezing, hives, or other allergic reactions.

Mary told me that, for years, she had a passion for yard work, lawn care, and gardening. She'd used fertilizers and other chemicals to ensure that her lawn was the envy of the neighborhood. As she talked, I learned that her sensitivities to multiple products began in the last dozen or so years and coincided with her retirement as a teacher and her growing interest in her yard.

I arranged for her to be tested for levels of solvents, pesticides, and other pollutants in her urine.

She was off the chart, so I referred her to a naturopathic doctor who worked in environmental toxins and poisons. He developed a program that helped Mary's body build up its liver detoxification pathways and antioxidant stores. He also treated her GI tract with botanicals and supplements that healed her leaky gut. He then had her detox with infrared sauna therapy, chlorella algae powders, and modified citrus pectin tablets. When Mary was tested a year later, her levels of toxins were dramatically lower and her sensitivity to perfumes and other agents had nearly resolved. And by the way, her advanced arterial testing was normal. Her quality of life and social connections had improved tremendously.

painting or when you've just brought home new furniture, mattresses, or other household items that might be emitting fumes. High-quality HEPA air filters are another option.

There are a lot of other things you can do to reduce indoor air pollution. Here are some ideas:

* **Look into organic furniture and mattresses.** Some of these might even be covered by your insurance as long as your physician writes a prescription for them.

* **Don't use air fresheners or paraffin candles.** If you want to improve the scent of your home, put some dried coffee grounds in a bowl, and set the bowl near any offending odors. The coffee will absorb the scent, so it's a natural deodorizer.

* **Get a dehumidifier.** High humidity levels increase the concentrations of some pollutants. Aim to keep humidity levels below 50 percent.

* **If your eyes burn, back off.** Think of your eyes as the canary in the coal mine. If they burn, then you are definitely around invisible fumes that could be harming your health. Inspect your surroundings for sources of irritation from gas leaks, solvents, or poor-quality air.

* **Keep houseplants.** They might help to naturally filter some of the fumes from the air. Just don't overwater them, as too-damp soil becomes a breeding group for microorganisms like mold and bacteria that can trigger allergies.

* **Use the exhaust fans in your kitchen and bathroom,** especially when cleaning, cooking, or otherwise using products that emit fumes into the air.

* **Keep containers of paint, kerosene, and other similar products outside of the house,** possibly in the garage

or shed. Fumes can leak from these cans once they've been opened, even if you've reattached the lid.

Power Rx: If You Exercise Outdoors, Do It in the Morning

The air pollution in Beijing, China, hovers around 500 particles per cubic meter of air. For some perspective, the U.S. Environmental Protection Agency advises all of us to curtail all outdoor activities whenever the smog count hits 300, and most U.S. cities consider their air to be dangerous when that count is much lower, in the neighborhood of 70 or 80.

Dangerous air quality became a problem during the 2008 Summer Olympics that were held in and around Beijing. Marathon runners, for example, inhale more than 10 times as much air as the average person. Not only would all that smog hurt their performances, it would create a lasting negative impact on their health.

In an attempt to reduce the smog count for a two-month period before and during the Olympics, administrators shut down factories, halted construction projects, and dramatically reduced the number of vehicles allowed to drive on the streets at any one time.

As China worked to lower the smog, an international team of researchers decided to take advantage of a unique situation. They knew that the smog in Beijing was likely to drop to an historic low during the games, but then rebound back to its worst after the games had ended, especially once China released all the restrictions on factories and traffic. The researchers wanted to know: How would this small window of relatively good air affect the health of people who lived in the city?

They decided to find out.

In the months before, during, and after the Olympics, the researchers took blood samples from Chinese medical residents. They also monitored blood pressure, heart rate, and other markers of health.

As expected, air pollution dropped during the games. Then it rebounded afterward, and when the researchers looked at the data, the implication was clear. In the months just before the games, when air pollution levels were lowest, blood samples showed less inflammation and blood-clotting proteins and lower blood pressure.

Heart attacks also decreased during this period.[134]

And after air pollution rose back to normal levels? Blood-clotting factors and blood pressure rose with it.

This is just one of thousands of studies that show the strong link between air pollution and heart health.[135]

The ozone, fine particulate matter, and carbon monoxide that form dirty air are as bad for your health as secondhand smoke. If you live in areas with more air pollution, or even just live closer to a highway, you have an increased risk for:

* Arterial plaque.
* Heart attacks.
* Strokes.
* Inflammation in the blood vessels.
* Thickened blood that is more likely to clot.
* Heart rate disturbances.

Rx at a Glance

No matter where you live, the cleanliness of your air will follow a predictable cycle. It will be cleanest between 6:00 a.m. and 10:00 a.m. That's because car exhaust and other forms of air pollution react with sunlight and heat. During the early morning, when the angle of the sun and the temperatures are lowest, you have a small window of cleaner air.

Because we inhale much more air during exercise than we do at rest, morning is the best time of day to exercise outdoors. Use this additional advice to reduce your exposure to pollutants:

* **Monitor your local air quality index as you monitor the weather.** You wouldn't power walk while chain-smoking, so don't walk, run, or cycle outdoors during a pollution alert, either.

* **Avoid exhaust fumes.** It may be just as dangerous for your health to run behind a car as it is to run in front of one. Exercise in a park, away from busy roadways. And while there's no true research to show it helps, I hold my breath for as long as possible when I am walking by a bus or truck spewing dark exhaust. It definitely can't hurt!

* **Stop exercising and get indoors.** If your lungs hurt or you have trouble breathing, it's a sign that you are gulping down dirty air.

Power Rx: If You Live in a City, Wear Noise-Cancelling Headphones

Many metropolitan areas are not only the most air-polluted places to live, but also the most noise-polluted.

And, as it turns out, noise pollution is almost as bad for your heart as smog.

Researchers analyzed data from a large population study on people who live in the Ruhr region of Germany, looking specifically at how air and noise pollution affected thoracic aortic calcification (TAC), a measure of hardening of the arteries. Detected with a simple chest X-ray, it provides an estimate of overall artery damage throughout the body. Calcium in an artery is always a sign of damage.

Air pollution caused TAC to spike by 20 percent, which should come as no surprise if you read the previous prescription about walking in the morning. Noise pollution caused the same health measure to shoot up by eight percent, and this was independent of the quality of the air on any given day.[136]

Previous research also found for every 10 decibels of noise from traffic, the risk of a heart attack is increased by 12 percent.[137]

How does noise contribute to hardening of the arteries? One mechanism might be stress. Even if you don't feel uncomfortable, noise might be setting off your fight-or-flight response and causing levels of stress hormones to rise. It also may simply cause an imbalance in the autonomic nervous system, which leads to increased blood pressure, blood lipids, blood glucose, and blood clotting.

Rx at a Glance

If you live in a city, you are surrounded by noise. It's so constant that you're probably not even aware of it. Use this advice:

* **Wear noise-cancelling headphones,** especially when on city sidewalks near high-traffic areas where there is a lot of noise. Use caution at intersections, of course.

* **Minimize your added noise exposure.** When traveling in a car, resist the urge to turn up the volume in an attempt to hear the radio over the sound of traffic.

* **Seek out quiet places.** Spend time in parks, churches, libraries, museums, and other areas where noise is lower.

Power Rx: Avoid Smoke

We have a word for someone who sits inside a running car in a closed garage: suicidal.

The same could be said of someone who sits next to a smoker in an enclosed room. Secondhand smoke contains 200 known poisons, including formaldehyde and carbon monoxide (the same poison that is emitted in car exhaust).

This form of air pollution not only contains 60 different carcinogens, it also contains countless blood vessel irritants. It ignites inflammation in the blood and arteries throughout the body, each year causing 50,000 heart disease deaths.[138]

Rx at a Glance

* **Don't smoke.** It's never too late to quit.

* **Don't stand next to anyone who is smoking.** Insist that smokers take it outside or quit, and avoid public sites where smoking is permitted.

* **Stay a safe distance from other forms of smoke,** such as fire pits and wood-burning stoves.

Power Rx: Don't Drink Petroleum (Ditch Plastic Water Bottles)

If I poured thick, black crude oil into a glass and asked you to drink it, you'd look at me as if I were crazy. You might even report me to the police.

Yet, I'm pretty sure, you are willingly drinking small amounts of petroleum every day in the form of plastic residue. All plastics are made from petroleum (made from crude oil), and plastic water bottles are no exception.

It would be nice if the plastic was self-contained and never leached into the water. Research shows, however, that this just isn't the case. A Saudi study of 10 different brands of bottled water found that plastic residue had leaked into every single one of them.[139] And a study from the *Journal of the American Medical Association* found that eating canned soup (from cans that had linings made from a type of plastic called bisphenol-A, or BPA) for five days raised urine levels of BPA 20 times compared to those of people who ate homemade soup.[140]

That means the water you drink from these bottles is laced with harmful chemicals such as bisphenol-A (BPA), bisphenol-S (BPS), and phthalates. Sometimes called endocrine disruptors because they interfere with the functioning of healthy hormones, these substances mimic the effects of estrogen, increasing your risk of prostate cancer, breast cancer, and obesity. And they may set the stage for heart disease, too. One study linked high blood levels of a certain type of phthalate metabolite to an increased risk of hardened, clogged arteries, and of BPA with an increased risk of dangerous types of plaque that are likely to rupture and cause sudden and often fatal heart attacks.[141]

These plastic residues are so pervasive that most of us already have measurable amounts in our bodies. Canada became the first country to label bisphenols a toxic substance in 2010, and recently the United States followed suit in terms of baby bottles, but not with other products.

Rx at a Glance

Whenever possible, don't drink from plastic containers. Instead of using plastic water bottles, outfit your sink with a water filter. When you must drink from a bottle, use this advice:

* **Use glass, porcelain, or stainless-steel water bottles rather than disposable plastic ones.**

* **If you must drink from a disposable container, use a paper cup rather than a plastic or Styrofoam one.**

* **If a plastic water bottle is your only option, don't freeze it and don't leave it sitting out in the sun.** The Saudi study I mentioned earlier found that both heat and extreme cold cause the plastic to break down, leaching more plastic residue into the water.[142]

* **If you must use a plastic bottle, choose wisely.** Bottles marked with recycle code 7 are the most likely to contain BPA and should be avoided. Codes 3 and 6 should be avoided as well. Codes 1, 2, 4, and 5 are less likely to contain toxins.

Power Rx: Make Your Kitchen a Plastic-Free Zone

Plastic water bottles are not the only source of bisphenol-A (BPA), bisphenol-S (BPS), and phthalates. Another common one: the plastic containers we use to transport, cook, and store our food.

BPA is used widely in plastic bottles, linings of food cans, and food storage containers. This plastic residue can leach into the food you eat. If your levels of BPA rise high enough, your hormonal system is thrown off.[143] Heart disease, nerve problems, sexual difficulties, cancer, obesity, and premature puberty are among the many health problems associated with bisphenol exposure.

When researchers from a number of different institutions looked at the levels of BPA in the urine of nearly 1,600 Brits and followed their health outcomes for 10 years, they found that people who developed heart disease were more likely to have elevated levels of BPA in their urine.[144] Research done in the United States by the same research team arrived at similar findings.[145]

Rx at a Glance

Think of plastic in much the same way you think of an old lover who caused you a lot of pain. Yes, you might still be attracted to it, but it's just not good for you. So keep your distance:

* **Use glass, ceramic, terra-cotta, and stainless storage containers instead of rubber and plastic,** especially when storing cheeses, meats, and tomato-based foods, since plastic is most likely to migrate into acidic and fatty foods.

* **Never microwave any food while it's in a plastic container.** If you wish to microwave a frozen dinner, remove the food from the container before microwaving it and nuke it on a plate or in a bowl.

* **Don't use steam-in-a-bag or boil-in-a-bag products.** Always remove foods from their plastic containers before cooking.

* **Use paper bags instead of plastic ones to transport foods.**

* **If you must use plastics in the kitchen, be sure they are labeled dishwasher and microwave safe.**

* **Look for BPA-free cans when buying beans and other canned items.** Muir Glen and Eden Foods now offer them, and other brands are quickly following their lead. If you can't find a BPA-free canned product, purchase the frozen version instead.

* **Don't use nonstick cookware.** Use glass, stainless, or cast iron instead.

* **Use wooden cooking utensils instead of plastic ones.**

* **Try a bamboo cutting board.** It's naturally antimicrobial, and won't leach plastic into your food.

* **Buy products in glass, paper, or cardboard containers** rather than plastic containers, if you can.

Power Rx: Don't Put Anything on Your Skin That You Wouldn't Eat

Our skin is our largest organ, and many people think of their skin in much the same way they think of Fort Knox: impenetrable. Yet this outer protective layer of our bodies is no such thing.

The outer layer of skin, called the stratum corneum, consists of tightly bound cells. Between each cell is a tiny space that is filled with fats, oils, and waxes. These spaces are so small that we can't see them with the naked eye, but they are large enough for some substances to slip through. Certain substances can even seep directly into the cells themselves. Either way, they eventually make their way into the bloodstream.

In many ways, this is beneficial. These tiny modes of entry are what allow medicinal patches—such as the birth control patch and the nicotine patch—to work their magic.

But these tiny entry points can also allow harmful substances into the body.

Think about all of the substances you put on your skin: sunscreen, bug spray, makeup, body lotion. Would you eat any of these substances? I'm guessing the answer is no, and it's not just because they would put a bad taste in your mouth.

The Environmental Working Group (www.ewg.org) estimates that the average woman uses 12 products containing 168 different chemicals every single day. Not all of these chemicals are harmful, and not all are capable of seeping through the skin, either, but some are. Among the most pervasive: phthalates.

These chemicals are used to soften many personal care products like perfumes, eye shadow, deodorant, insect repellent, moisturizers, nail polish, liquid soap, and hair spray. They are easily absorbed into the body. Phthalates act as endocrine disruptors (like BPA, which is also found in many personal care products) and may play a role in obesity, thyroid disease, and even some cancers. Recently, high blood pressure in children has been linked to phthalate exposures. More than 50 medical papers link phthalates to cardiovascular issues.

There are many different kinds of phthalates, some of which are banned by the European Union because they are so destructive to human health. Canada heavily regulates their use, keeping them to a minimum in children's toys and children's care products.

But they are not banned in the United States, and the cosmetic industry is not regulated. So you can assume that they are probably in most of the creams, makeup, and other products you put on your body every day. What else is in these products? Many also contain parabens (a possible carcinogen and endocrine disruptor) and xylene (an irritant that depresses the nervous system). Mercury has been found in some mascaras. And an FDA analysis found lead in several popular brands of lipstick, including certain types by Maybelline, L'Oreal, Cover Girl, Revlon, and even Burt's Bees.[146]

These chemicals are so pervasive that, when the Environmental Working Group tested teen girls, they found 16 different chemicals from cosmetics had leeched into their bodies, including phthalates, triclosan (an ingredient added to many consumer products that is currently under FDA review for possible health-harming effects), and parabens—which showed up in their blood and urine samples.[147]

Rx at a Glance

If you wouldn't eat it, why would you put it on your body? There are plenty of good-for-you edible substances that can perform the same functions as many of these plastic-infused personal care products.

* **For moisturizer:** Use olive, almond, coconut, or another natural oil.

* **For makeup:** Use blush, foundation, and eye shadow made from minerals, a type of makeup that is becoming increasingly more available and mainstream.

* **For an anti-aging and beauty cream:** You can find many natural recipes all over the Internet. Try two egg whites mixed with 2 tablespoons of yogurt or a mixture of ½ cup pumpkin pulp, 2 teaspoons almond milk, 1 teaspoon honey, and 2 teaspoons cranberry juice for starters.

* **For soap:** Make a sugar scrub from sugar, water, and a natural oil.

Sometimes the health reasons for putting chemicals onto our skin outweigh the health reasons against doing so. For instance, melanoma is a deadly form of skin cancer that develops on skin exposed to the sun. While staying out of excessive sun is key, it's not always an option. When you have to be in the sun, sunscreen is a must, but use great care in picking a sunscreen. When the Environmental Working Group examined 500 types of sunscreens, fewer than 50 brands were endorsed as safe. Visit their website to follow their recommendations.

Power Rx: Study Ingredient Labels Like Jane Goodall Studies Chimps

If you are experiencing a bit of déjà vu, it's for good reason. Yes, you found similar advice in the Nutrition Rx section on page 100. In that chapter, however, I was talking about food labels. Here, I'm talking about household products.

You will hopefully be able to follow the previous prescription—"Don't Put Anything On Your Skin That You Wouldn't Eat"—at least some of the time. Chances are, however, you won't be able to do it for every single household product. In some cases, a real-food alternative just may not exist. In other cases, you may be unwilling to spend the time making it yourself. I get it.

That's why label reading is so important. Don't trust any packaging claims that state that the product is "dermatologist tested" or "hypoallergenic." Always read the label, and take any listed warnings very seriously.

Rx at a Glance

If you are a good sleuth, you'll be able to avoid using toothpastes, soaps, deodorants, mouthwashes, and cosmetics that contain the following harmful ingredients:

* **Triclosan and triclocarban.**
* **Triethanolamine (TEA).**
* **DMDM hydantoin.**
* **Imidazolidinyl urea.**
* **Fragrances and dyes.**
* **Parabens.**
* **Sodium lauryl sulfate or sodium laureth sulfate.**
* **Oxybenzone.**

If you're unsure whether a product is safe, consult the Environmental Working Group's www.ewg.org/skindeep/, which offers a safety rating on many brands.

Power Rx: Clean with Food, Not with Chemicals

Perhaps you are noticing a trend. Not only are self-care products laced with harmful chemicals, so are many cleaning products. These are often called persistent organic pollutants (POPS) and have been linked to strokes, heart disease, high blood pressure, and artery damage. Among the dangerous heart-harming ingredients:

Volatile organic compounds. These are the same dangerous substances in smog, and they contribute to respiratory problems, headaches, and allergies.

Formaldehyde. This colorless gas is used as a disinfectant. It's a carcinogen that can pass through the skin and also be inhaled, irritating the lungs. Since there is no safe level, it's best to reduce your exposure as much as possible.

Phthalates. Sound familiar? Yes, these endocrine disruptors are found in any cleaning product that produces a "fresh clean scent."

Triclosan. This antibacterial agent is another endocrine disruptor. If you have antibacterial hand soap at home or work, odds are it has triclosan in it. I would recommend ditching it.

Rx at a Glance

Whenever possible, clean with items that you wouldn't mind adding to any dish you cook in the kitchen: baking soda, lemon, white vinegar, alcohol, and cornstarch. Also, use this advice:

* **Don't be duped by marketing claims that the products are "green."** That doesn't mean they are safer. Check

the list of ingredients to see what the product actually contains. If you see words like "vinegar," "peppermint," and "lemon juice," you're probably in the clear. If you see words like "colorant" and "fragrance," chances are you are not.

* **Don't use air fresheners at all.** The chemicals in air fresheners can react with ozone to form formaldehyde and other dangerous particles.[148] Use coffee grounds or another natural alternative.

* **When using any cleaning product, open the windows to keep the air circulating.**

* **Try these easy swaps:** a rag soaked with tea instead of furniture polish, ketchup instead of copper cleaner, kosher or sea salt instead of oven cleaner or a stain remover, vodka instead of tile and window cleaner.

Power Rx: Air Out Your Dry Cleaning

How exactly does a dry cleaner get those stains out of your clothes? You guessed it: with chemicals. They use liquid solvents to remove most of the stains, and one of these solvents is a clear, colorless liquid with a sharp, sweet odor: perchloroethylene, or "perc."

Perc is great at removing stains. It also protects clothes against shrinking, it evaporates quickly, and it can be reused over and over again, making it very cost effective. That's why as many as 85 percent of dry cleaners use it as their primary solvent. But it comes at a price.

These solvents have been detected in random blood and urine samples, and may be a cause of chronic illnesses that defy explanation. Exposure to this chemical results in dizziness, fatigue, headaches, and nausea. It has been shown to cause cancer in rats and mice and is rated "probably carcinogenic to humans" by the International Agency for Research on Cancer (IARC). The relationship to heart disease is not yet certain, but the toxic effect of perc on important enzyme systems including the liver is concerning, and it's something I take very seriously.

Rx at a Glance

This doesn't mean you must shun the dry cleaners, but it's wise to take some precautions:

* **When you come home with the dry cleaning, remove the plastic wrap and let your clothes hang in the garage or somewhere else outside of your living space** for a few days so they can de-gas.

* **Also, look for a green dry cleaner.** In recent years, some dry cleaners have found ways to reduce their use of perc, but the Environmental Protection Agency estimates that at least 85 percent of dry cleaners are still using it as their primary solvent. Try to find one of the 15 percent that does not.

Power Rx: Keep Your Phone at Arm's Length

Every time I perform an electrocardiogram (ECG), which measures changes in the heart's electrical currents, I am reminded that our bodies are energetic structures. Every heartbeat is due to waves of electrical current.

This is why it's worth considering how new technologies, including cell phones, affect the function of our cells. Without a doubt, cell phones can save lives. They enable quicker notification of emergency medical services, speed up transmission of medical records, and expedite the recording of an ECG for rhythm analysis.

But we should be worried about how cell phones affect the function of the heart, especially because so many of us carry these gadgets in our pocket right over our ticker.

Here's what we know: Electromagnetic energy emitted by cell

phones appears to increase reactive oxygen species (oxidation or rust, a common mechanism of aging and disease), weaken cell membranes, and alter the handling of calcium in cells. It might also damage the DNA in our mitochondria, the powerhouse of all cells for energy production.

In a recent study of Indian medical students, a one-minute phone call raised the heart rate in chronic users of cell phones. The blood cholesterol levels were also higher in regular users.[149] A separate study found a relationship between cell phone use and a harmful disturbance in heart rate variability.[150]

Of more concern is a study of patients with clogged arteries. Over 100 of these patients had an ECG performed while a cell phone in the off position was placed at their waist and then over their heart. Then the ECG was repeated while the phone rang for 40 seconds at the same positions. The cell phone ring over the heart caused more heart rhythm disturbances than when it was at their waist.[151]

In 1996, the FCC established limits for safe exposure to radio frequency energy based on a measurement called the Specific Absorption Rate (SAR). A man with a large body frame and head size would reach the SAR limits after talking on his cell phone for just six minutes a day. Most of us now talk on our cell phones much more than that—the average daily use exceeds 30 minutes. And presumably, smaller-framed men, women, and children would reach the limits faster.

Plus, the farther you are from the nearest cell tower, the more energy your phone needs to emit to get a signal. Same goes if you're in a car or a building. Your phone's energy output also surges when you switch from cell tower to cell tower, as you do when you're walking or driving while on your phone.

Rx at a Glance

The science on cell phone safety is still emerging and, at this point, our gaps of knowledge are great. So the best advice I can give you is to follow the advice of your cell phone manufacturer, the very advice you probably neglected to read in the legal statement of your owner's guide. Apple, the maker of my iPhone, includes a legal statement that states that you should "carry the iPhone at least 10 mm away from your body to ensure exposure levels remain at or below the as-tested levels."

So keep your distance. Also, use your phone as sparingly as possible. And as we wait for the research to come in, the following advice is probably wise:

* **Avoid carrying a cell phone in your bra or in your left front pocket over your heart.** Instead, carry it as far away as you can, preferably in a purse, briefcase, or bag. And, yes, many women carry their phone in their bra. I have seen it hundreds of times, especially at the gym.

* **Embrace texting.** Phones emit less radiation when you send a text than when you make a call.

* **Put your phone in airplane mode whenever you can.** This turns off the signal on the phone, stopping it from trying to connect with cell towers and reducing the radiation exposure.

* **Don't talk when you only have half a bar.** Not only will the dropped calls and bad connection fill you with anxiety and negativity, the weak signal may also increase emissions from your cell phone antenna.

* **Use a headset whenever possible to increase your distance from the phone.** This allows you to talk with the phone farther away from your body, reducing your exposure.

YOUR FINAL ECO RX

Have I scared you into selling your home and moving back to the woods with a dial phone and lard soap? I hope not. You can still live a modern existence—with all its conveniences. You just need to be very careful about the products you put in your home and on your body.

As with previous chapters, start with any prescription that seems most realistic to you and break it down into small steps. Maybe next time you are at the grocery store, you carefully read labels for toothpaste and a few other products. The next time you need to polish your dining room table would be a great time to try polishing that wood with a tea-soaked cloth rather than furniture polish. And when you walk into a room and realize that your pet has made it smell like a frat house, get out the coffee grounds.

It's small changes, done consistently over time, that add up to big results. So don't overwhelm yourself. Go slowly, and incorporate more and more prescriptions over time.

This process might become easier in the years ahead. The Environmental Protection Agency is working to limit our exposure to the most toxic of known chemicals. They have called for a global effort to reduce these toxins, and an international agreement in 2001 of the Stockholm Convention has made a difference. They target POPS that can be transported by wind or water across continents and seek to ban them. They have published the names of a dirty dozen of POPS, including DDT, PCBs, dioxins, and others. The United States is not yet a party to the convention, but has signed an agreement with Canada to eliminate POPS in the Great Lakes Region.

In the meantime, buyers beware. Read the labels, visit a health food store in your area that carries personal and home cleaning items, avoid nonstick cookware, and ask questions.

Two great resources that will help you in your quest:

The Environmental Working Group contains an extensive database that ranks hundreds of consumer products for safety (www.ewg.org).

ConsumerLab.com tests various consumer products to make sure they contain the active ingredients they advertise and that they don't contain harmful ingredients like lead.

Chapter 11

Your Supplement Rx

I got interested in supplements when I began searching for ways to help my patients with congestive heart failure. This is a condition characterized by shortness of breath and tissue swelling that prompts many people to go to the hospital and can even lead to death if not treated promptly. I was troubled that despite many prescription medications, many of my patients were having their lives cut short.

I went back to my medical school biochemistry textbooks. Over and over again, one fact kept coming to my attention: Energy production, or ATP, was what heart cells needed most. And Coenzyme Q10 (CoQ10) was repeatedly mentioned as a factor in producing ATP. This led me to look into the work of a leader of integrative cardiology, Dr. Stephen Sinatra.

I read his papers and books and, as a result, began suggesting supplements as well as prescription medications for my patients with congestive heart failure. Once I did so, my patients reported better energy, fewer problems, and fewer trips to the emergency room. I have since treated thousands of patients with a combination of supplements, all targeted to optimize the function of their mitochondria inside their heart cells. Lesson learned: Medical

Ask the Holistic Heart Doc:

I've heard of chelation therapy. Is this something I should consider?

What is chelation? The therapy involves oral or intravenous medicines that bind to heavy metals and even minerals such as the calcium in your arteries, sweeping toxins and artery-narrowing plaque away and eventually to your kidneys, which sweep it out of your body in your urine. In some people this can be lifesaving because heavy metals such as lead, mercury, and cadmium can accumulate in the heart and its arteries, poisoning enzymes and damaging the heart.

For many years, this therapy was shunned by standard practitioners due to an absence of research data. More recently, however, the U.S. government's National Institutes of Health funded a study of more than 1,700 heart attack survivors, the Trial to Assess Chelation Therapy (TACT). Published in the prestigious *Journal of the American Medical Association,* this study found that chelation therapy reduced cardiac events such as heart attack by 18 percent compared to patients who didn't receive the therapy. Study participants who had diabetes experienced even more dramatic results: a stunning 39 percent drop in cardiac events.[152]

Chelation isn't for everyone, but it can be especially helpful if you are suffering the effects of toxic overload from smoking, dental fillings, or environmental exposure (for instance, if your job required you to work in an area later found to be contaminated by lead). To determine whether the therapy is right for you, your health care provider will test your urine, blood, or possibly even hair for toxins.

I've recommended this therapy to a few patients, and the results have been encouraging. Unfortunately, insurance does not yet cover chelation therapy for heart disease, so most patients have to pay for the weekly sessions out of pocket. Depending on the severity of your toxic overload, you'll need anywhere from five to 30 treatments, spanning several months to even over a year, and the costs can run well over $1,000.

professionals can improve the supply of oxygen to the heart and other organs by stents, bypass, and unique treatments like external counterpulsation, but if the factors to produce energy in the cell are deficient, the results are rarely optimal.

From there, I moved on to study supplements that aid antioxidant function, liver detoxification, methylation, and arterial function. Although research shows that a whole food, plant-based, organic diet is the most effective way to improve mitochondrial function and produce energy in the heart cells, at a time that the nutrition we get from our food is dropping rapidly and our world is more toxic than ever before, I strongly believe that a reasonable recommendation for the use of vitamins and supplements is needed. And yes, I take them myself.

Yet few topics in the medical world divide health professionals more.

Recently, a prominent professor from a major university lectured at my hospital during grand rounds for residents and students. This professor has published many research articles and books about treating high blood pressure with nutrition and vitamins. During the lecture, he reviewed his own original published research and that of others around the world. At the end of his wonderful presentation, the chief of medicine of our hospital stood up. I, along with many others in the room, assumed that he was about to thank and congratulate the guest speaker. Instead, he warned the medical students and residents that everything the prominent professor had said was just conjecture and should never be tried in the hospital on any patients!

Why is there so much disagreement? Primarily it's because the research isn't conclusive. There are hundreds of small, medium, and even large studies that demonstrate health benefits for various supplements. At the same time, there are articles that show no benefit, and a few that show harm. This has led some to declare supplements "useless." Some even say they are dangerous, causing the very diseases they are being taken to prevent.

How could some studies find a benefit while others found no

effect and still others link supplements with poor health? Let's take a closer look at all the varied reasons why so many studies might arrive at such opposing findings:

Scientists don't always study the best supplements. Not all supplements are created equally. That's because some are made from real foods and some are made synthetically. Some come from companies with tight quality controls, ensuring that the actual active ingredients are inside of every single pill. Others come from companies without these controls, so what's actually inside the pill or capsule is not necessarily what's claimed on the bottle. Perhaps most important, there are many different varieties of most vitamins and minerals. For instance, if you check various supplement bottles at the store, you'll find two types of vitamin D (D_2 and D_3), four types of calcium (carbonate, citrate, gluconate, and lactate) and eight types of vitamin E (alpha-, beta-, gamma-, and delta-tocopherol and alpha-, beta-, gamma-, and delta-tocotrienol).

Some of these varieties are much more effective than others. Let's talk about vitamin E specifically. Some studies show that this vitamin helps block the unhealthy LDL cholesterol from oxidizing and damaging the arteries, prevent heart disease, and reduce dangerous blood clots. But other studies found no benefit. How could this be? The studies that failed to find a benefit used only one type of vitamin E (not a range of four to eight types as is found in nature), used synthetic sources, and studied only alpha-tocopherol. High doses of alpha-tocopherol may block the effects of the other types of vitamin E such as gamma-tocopherol and promote, not block, oxidation. In nature and in plant-based, whole foods, vitamins don't exist in isolation but come combined to provide a spectrum of balanced actions.

Scientists often look at supplements through a reductionist microscope. The trend in medicine is to reduce science to a single focus, the so-called reductionist philosophy of René Descartes. Sometimes a single focus bears fruit. A single antibiotic was found to heal pneumonia. Other times, however, an army of treatments is needed to cure or reverse disease. Many studies have examined a single supplement and found that it did not prevent or heal a disease. That finding might be correct. But it's also possible that a few different supplements need to work together to prevent or heal disease.

In some supplement studies, no blood tests were performed. Blood levels of omega-3 fatty acids, vitamin D, and CoQ10 are easy to study, but few of the headline studies have measured these. This is important because, as I said, not all companies have the best quality control measures in place. Also, it's hard to say whether another factor—ranging from a prescription medicine to the health of the subject's GI tract—could block absorption of a supplement. So, in some studies, it's possible that the reason participants didn't benefit from taking a supplement was because their bodies didn't absorb it, not because the vitamin or other nutrient in the supplement doesn't help.

Studies are not all done in the same way. It's not easy to compare the results of one study to another and arrive at any conclusion. Different studies test different doses of vitamins for different lengths of time. Take vitamin D as an example. Studies have found that it protects against fractures at doses of 700 to 800 IU a day, but that 400 IU a day has less benefit. A short vitamin supplement trial may not show any benefit simply because it takes a long time for a disease to develop or for the vitamin's protective effects to emerge. Similarly, the study population might matter, too. A supplement is most useful on the population of people who need it for health reasons or who are deficient in it. A trial done on smokers will reveal different results than a trial done on marathoners, which will also arrive at different results than a trial done on vegans.

Most supplements are not patented. You can't patent a product found in the human body unless the delivery mechanism itself can be patented. Therefore, the number of high-quality, pharmaceutical-grade vitamin providers is small and represents a tiny fraction of supplements that are studied. Most studies of supplements are also small due to limited funding.

WHAT THE NAYSAYERS ARE RIGHT ABOUT

There are some truths when it comes to nutritional supplements, truths that my colleagues and I agree on.

Truth #1: Plant foods are nature's miracles. No human-made substance will ever be able to copy and package their goodness. Many foods come packaged with thousands of substances that protect against diseases, help your body absorb other important substances, and work together synergistically. An orange, for example, provides vitamin C, beta-carotene, calcium, fiber, water, and many phytochemicals. These nutrients might work together inside the human body. Isolating them might cause them to lose some of their power. This is why the lycopene from tomatoes offers more of a benefit than a lycopene supplement.

Truth #2: Plant foods contain countless healing nutrients, and we've only discovered and studied a small fraction of them. It's possible that, for instance, vitamin C isn't the most powerfully healing substance found in an orange. Maybe there's also a substance in those orange, juicy balls that's 100 times more powerful. We just don't know because we haven't discovered it yet.

Truth #3: Not all supplements are needed. Some are overhyped. Others don't contain what the bottle claims, and, yes, some might be dangerous, especially when taken in high amounts because of contaminants introduced with sloppy production.

Truth #4: *Taking supplements in an effort to counteract an unhealthy diet is like wearing a seat belt while you are in a car with a drunk driver behind the wheel.* The basis of good nutrition remains a plate loaded with colorful vegetables and fruits and accented with nuts, seeds, and beans. Processed foods, artificial sweeteners, and partially hydrogenated vegetable oils are best avoided. This isn't an either/or. Eat a diet full of wholesome, plant-based foods (as described in Chapter 6) and take the supplements described in this chapter. Don't use supplements as a Band-aid for an unhealthy diet.

WHY YOU MIGHT NEED SUPPLEMENTS

I firmly believe that certain supplements are not only good for you, but they are absolutely essential. Skip them and it's like skipping an important medicine prescribed by your health care provider.

In fact, the only difference between many supplements and many medicines is this: You need a health care provider to write a prescription for medicine. You don't for a supplement. Consider that digoxin, a potent prescription heart drug, comes from a plant: foxglove (also called digitalis). Similarly, aspirin comes from willow tree bark. One requires a prescription. The other does not. Both offer health benefits in the proper setting.

Why might additional supplements ever be needed? Why do I take supplements when my diet is plant-strong, vegan, and organic? There are at least six important reasons:

Our soil isn't as rich as it once was. Big corporate farming practices have depleted the soil of essential nutrients, so veggies and fruits don't contain as much nutrition as they did 50 or more years ago. A bowl of spinach now may look the same but when measured, it contains nearly 50 percent lower levels of iron, vitamin C, and other nutrients, compared to historical measurements.[153] You might have to eat three, four, or even five bowlfuls of spinach to match one from your grandparents' time.

We're living longer than ever before. While this is generally a good thing, our bodies don't work as well as we age. People older than age 50, for instance, benefit from B_{12} supplementation because absorption of this vitamin in the digestive tract becomes less efficient with age.

There's a difference between "getting by" and "living optimally." The government's recommended daily allowances may be high enough to help you avoid a disease, such as scurvy, but they are too low, in many cases, to promote "optimal" functioning and health, particularly when there is a disease state already present.

Your medicines deplete your body. The very prescription medicines you might need to treat existing heart disease (and other common conditions) could increase your need for certain vitamins and minerals. The list of medications that may deplete important nutrients or hormones in the body is rather long. For example, statins—medicines used to lower blood cholesterol and soothe inflammation—deplete vitamins D and E, zinc, carnitine, selenium, and testosterone. Some cholesterol-lowering medications, like fenofibrate, can deplete vitamin B_{12}, vitamin E, copper, and zinc. Digoxin can deplete magnesium. Metformin, used for diabetes and polycystic ovarian disease, can deplete vitamin B_{12} and perhaps CoQ10. Drugs used for acid reflux like proton pump inhibitors can deplete vitamins D and B_{12} and have been linked to bone loss and osteoporosis. Finally, H2 receptor blockers like cimetidine (also used for reflux disease and heartburn) can also deplete vitamins B_{12} and D, zinc, folate, calcium, and iron. It is no wonder why I discover so many nutrient deficiencies in my patients.

Our lifestyles make us deficient in some nutrients. The best example of this is vitamin D. We need sunlight for our skin to make this important vitamin. But ever since our toxic lifestyles burned a hole in the ozone layer, we've all had to lather on sunscreen to avoid getting skin cancer. As a result, more people than ever are deficient in vitamin D.

Another example has to do with the organisms that live in our guts. Modern farming practices dose animals with low levels of antibiotics on a regular basis, and these antibiotics get into our bodies when we eat these animals. Among other things, they continually wipe out some of our good gut bacteria, necessitating the need for probiotic supplements, which resupply our intestines with helpful bacteria.

Not everyone eats the healthiest foods. Let's face it, many of us don't eat the best nature has to offer at every single eating opportunity. Even I have fallen victim to the lure of lunch on the run as I've rushed from the hospital to my office. If I am really in a pinch, I will very occasionally pull into a Burger King, the only national chain with a drive-thru that has a veggie burger. Once every few months, this "less junkie than most junk food" choice on a white bun might pass my lips, usually with the bun and sauces removed. The anemic piece of iceberg lettuce and a thin slice of tomato are a small nod to plant-based eating. Mea culpa.

Power Rx: Do a Background Check on Your Supplements

If you are already taking supplements, go get the bottles now. Do you know what's actually in those bottles? Do they contain the active ingredient claimed on the label? Is it possible that they house harmful heavy metals or other contaminants?

The answers to those questions will probably surprise you. Some of them probably don't contain what they claim. Others might offer much more than you ever wanted.

The sad truth is that the supplement industry is not regulated in the same way as the food industry or the prescription medicine industry. As a result, you can't always trust the manufacturer.

ConsumerLab.com has been testing health and nutrition products for many years, and, for a die-hard supplement fan like myself, their results have been a bit sobering. Consider these recent findings that came to light even as I was putting the finishing touches on this book:

* 31 percent of protein powders include more carbohydrate than they do protein.[154]

* The caffeine and catechin levels in bottled green tea products vary by as much as 240 percent, and some contain significant amounts of lead.[155]

* Some brands of Coenzyme Q10 (a supplement that I highly recommend) contain only 3.8 percent of the amount they claim in their labels.[156]

* Popular brands of vitamin D (another vitamin I highly recommend) and calcium failed to break apart, possibly preventing them from being absorbed into the body.[157]

Rx at a Glance

For all of the supplements you are currently taking along with all that you purchase in the future, always do a background check, using these guidelines.

* **Check with ConsumerLab.com to see if they have done a study on the types of supplements you are taking.** You must buy a membership with ConsumerLab in order to do so, but it's worth it. I am not a shill for the company. I only believe in what it has to offer.

* **Look for independent organizations that offer "seals of approval" that may be displayed on certain dietary supplement products.** These indicate that the product has passed the organization's quality tests for things such as potency and contaminants. These "seals of approval" do not mean that the product is safe or effective, but they do provide assurance that the product was properly manufactured, that it contains the ingredients listed on the label, and that it does not contain harmful levels of contaminants. Look for seals of approval from ConsumerLab.com, the National Science Foundation's Good Manufacturing Practices stamp, or the U.S. Pharmacopeia (USP) dietary supplement verification mark.

Power Rx: Take Natural Multivitamins

A daily multivitamin is your best insurance against nutrient deficiency, and various studies show that it also might be your best chance at avoiding a premature death.

A trial known as the TACT study (Trial to Assess Chelation Therapy), gave study participants IV or oral chelation therapy in the hopes of removing toxins and heavy metals from their arteries and therefore reducing blockages. The U.S. government sponsored the study of more than 1,700 survivors of a heart attack. Half got the IV therapy for over a year and the other half got a placebo.

In the second part of this study, half of the patients got a potent natural multivitamin requiring three capsules in the morning and three in the evening. Others got a placebo. Whom do you think had the lowest incidence of cardiac events like heart attack, hospitalization, and death? You're right. It was the patients who took the high-potency multivitamins before two meals rather than the ones who took the placebos.[158]

Remember that not all multivitamins are the same. The cheap ones that you buy at the drugstore are probably made from synthetic ingredients and may even contain plastic residue. Many of them contain too much of some nutrients and not enough of others—possibly even none of the most important ones for heart health.

So consider replacing the synthetic multivitamin you might have bought at the drugstore with natural multivitamins, made from real food ingredients.

Rx at a Glance

Over the years, I've tried many different brands of multivitamins, read many different labels, and researched the available studies. There are a few that I recommend often and take myself. They are Life Extension, Garden of Life, Orthomolecular Products, Metagenics, Biotics Research Corporation, XYMOGEN, Thorne, and the supplement labels for Dr. Joel Fuhrman, Dr. Joseph Mercola, and Dr. Stephen Sinatra. If you can find those brands, I recommend you stick with them. If not, when shopping for a multivitamin, use these guidelines:

* **Avoid retinol, retinyl palmitate, and retinyl acetate,** which may increase the risk of hip fracture and certain birth defects when taken at levels exceeding 10,000 IUs.

Natalie's Journey to a Lasting Heart

I liked Natalie and her husband Paul right away. Unfortunately, I met them both in the emergency room of a local hospital, soon after Natalie had come in complaining of shortness of breath. Tests done at the hospital revealed leaky heart valves, blocked heart arteries, and a weakened heart. It was serious.

She underwent bypass surgery with valve repair, but her recovery was suboptimal despite the best of medications. Several months later, she still remained short of breath due to her weakened heart, and had to cut back on many activities. Her love for her grandchildren kept her searching for options to feel more energetic.

I started her on a program of CoQ10, L-carnitine, D-ribose, and magnesium. Natalie at first balked at the additional pills and powders. I suggested she dump some of the supplements in a blender and make a smoothie to make it easier to get them all down. She did great with this plan.

Within just two months, she had more energy. At that point I added a fifth supplement for the heart, taurine, which often acts as a natural diuretic (water pill). This tweak to her regimen worked like a charm. Natalie came to her next office visit with a bounce in her step. Her quality of life has vastly improved. She says two supplement-packed smoothies a day is a small price to pay for good health. And recently, more than five years since her cardiac surgery, a follow-up test of her heart function shows that it has dramatically improved and is nearing normal. That's not bad for a few dollars a day of vitamins she buys at the shop a mile from her house.

* **Look for all-natural multivitamins derived from actual food sources** so the body can absorb a much larger percentage of their nutrients. Many multivitamins contain synthetic nutrients instead of natural ones, which are harder for the body to absorb.

* **If you are a man or a postmenopausal woman, avoid taking multivitamins that contain 18 mg or more of iron** (unless otherwise specified by your health care provider). Iron can collect in body tissues and organs, such as the liver and heart, and damage them.

* **If you take medicine to reduce blood clotting, such as warfarin (Coumadin and other brand names), see if your multivitamin contains vitamin K.** Vitamin K lowers the effectiveness of these drugs. Your health care provider can base the medicine dose partly on the amount of vitamin K you usually consume in foods and supplements.

* **Take the right E.** Most multivitamins only have one type of vitamin E, from a synthetic source. The risk of prostate cancer is actually higher if you take racemic alpha-tocopherol acetate, a version of vitamin E that is found in many inexpensive preparations. I would not permit this form of vitamin E in my body! A better choice is a supplement with mixed vitamin E preparations, including tocopherols and tocotrienols from natural sources like annattto, rice, or palm oils.

Power Rx: Buy Supplements from Trusted Sources

Many of the vitamins found in wholesale discount stores, local drugstores, and grocery stores are made from synthetic materials that are often based on petrochemicals, not fruits, vegetables, and other whole foods.

In Chapter 10, I mentioned phthalates, plastic toxins that have infiltrated our food system. Remember: Not only do these toxins disrupt the endocrine system; they also raise the risk for heart disease.

Unfortunately for us, phthalates have also infiltrated our medical system. The toxic substances are used to line IV bags and medical tubing, and they are also used to make vitamins, supplements, and various prescription medications.

When researchers from Harvard and Boston universities studied over-the-counter and prescription drugs sold since 1995, more than 100 of the brands—10 to 20 percent of the total—contained phthalates.[159] They've been found in fish oil supplements and in garlic pills, slow-release tablets and probiotics, too. Because the Food and Drug Administration considers them "inactive," they don't have to be listed in the supplement ingredients.

Rx at a Glance

If your vitamins and your motor oil have a lot in common maybe you should rethink where and from whom you purchase your supplements! I like to buy my supplements from the producers I listed earlier because they have a track record of high quality and consistently earn high marks from ConsumerLab.com. In lieu of that brand, you can do the following:

* **Read the drug facts panel, under "inactive ingredients."** Look for two word phrases with phthalate as the second word, such as "diethyl phthalate" and "dibutyl phthalate." Abbreviations such as DEHP, DBP, DEP, DMP, HMP, PVAP, CAP, and PET all also suggest phthalates.

* **Be wary of brands labeled "enteric coated" and "time release."** These are especially likely to contain phthalates. If you see the words "fragrance" or "parfum," it also probably contains phthalates.

* **Talk to your pharmacist.** Sometimes he or she can help you find varieties that are phthalate free.

* **Research your favorite brands online.** What you can't find listed on the bottle you can sometimes find listed on the manufacturer website.

Power Rx: Take Coenzyme Q10 (CoQ10)

Especially important for vegetarians and anyone on a statin or who has existing heart disease, this supplement helps to keep heart muscle cells healthy.

Most of the heart is made up of muscle cells that contract and relax about 100,000 times a day to lift blood out of the heart and send it into the lungs for oxygen or throughout the body to provide the building blocks of cellular function. Inside each heart muscle cell is a part called the mitochondria. These special organelles are like factories, having long production lines to take raw materials like oxygen and nutrients, and produce energy used by the cells to perform this miracle of continual work.

Having healthy mitochondria is a key goal of heart disease prevention and treatment. The energy molecule that mitochondria produce is called ATP, or adenosine triphosphate. In conditions like angina pectoris (exertional chest pain due to blocked arteries), congestive heart failure, heart attacks, and cardiomyopathies (weakened heart muscles), levels of ATP in the cells are low. The cells have both used up their pool of ATP and produced too little. In fact, cells may store only enough ATP to power a heart cell for 10 seconds. If the machinery of the mitochondria is not humming at peak efficiency, heart health will falter. Coenzyme Q10 (CoQ10) is essential for the production of ATP. This agent both acts as a powerful antioxidant to fight the stresses and damage that oxygen-free radicals cause and is involved in the machinery of mitochondria to produce energy. So for optimal heart health, we want to make sure we have adequate levels of CoQ10. This supplement is especially important for:

Anyone with existing heart disease. Recent studies suggest that CoQ10 supplementation increases heart contraction, reduces complications of open-heart surgery, and lowers blood pressure and cholesterol. When more than 400 patients with advanced heart failure were given CoQ10 or a placebo, the CoQ10 group cut their risk of heart deaths in half. That's not bad for a supplement that can be purchased over the counter.

Anyone on a statin. As I mentioned earlier, statins reduce cholesterol by blocking an enzyme that contributes to cholesterol production. What else is blocked by statin drugs? The production of CoQ10! If you use statins, your CoQ10 levels might be 30 to 40 percent lower than normal.

Anyone over age 40. CoQ10 levels tend to decline with age. Vegetarians also tend to test low in this important coenzyme.

Rx at a Glance

Most heart patients are treated with 200 to 400 mg a day. If you are taking CoQ10, use these pointers:

* **Consider asking your health care provider to measure CoQ10 levels in your blood.** This will help you and your health care provider to pinpoint the optimal dose for you. CoQ10 levels in the blood should be over 3 µg/ml. If they remain lower, increase your supplemental dose from 200 mg a day to 400 mg a day, or to even 600 mg a day.

* **Combine it with selenium.** Selenium is a mineral that is also important for heart cells. In one study of healthy elderly people, CoQ10 plus selenium reduced the risk of death by over 50 percent.[160]

Power Rx: Try This Pill of Sunshine (Vitamin D)

I measure vitamin D blood levels in all my patients. Ninety-five percent of them test low. Even my medical friends practicing in sunny climates like Arizona tell me they find the same uniform deficiencies.

At the same time, data continues to accumulate showing that adequate vitamin D levels are necessary for the prevention of congestive heart failure and cancer, low levels of blood pressure and blood sugar, and the health of your brain and your bones.

Not long ago researchers from the University of Copenhagen and Copenhagen University Hospital found that people with low blood levels of D were at a much greater risk of developing heart disease than people with higher levels. In their study of more than 10,000 Danes, low levels of D were associated with a 40 percent greater risk of heart disease, a 64 percent greater risk of heart attack, and a 57 percent greater risk of early death.[161]

A separate study found that for every 10 percent more D people had in their blood, the risk of high blood pressure dropped by eight percent.[162]

Direct sunshine on exposed skin for 20 to 30 minutes a day can provide adequate vitamin D for some, but for most of us, oral supplementation is necessary. You probably need more D if:

You're a person of color. The darker your skin pigment, the harder it is for your skin to make D.

You're overweight. D gets trapped in fat cells. Once inside, it has a hard time getting back out.

You're vegan. Since fortified dairy is one of the main vitamin D food sources, vegans tend to be lower in D than nonvegans. Although mushrooms are a great source of D, I recommend all vegans take a D supplement, too.

Rx at a Glance

Take a supplement that contains 1,000 IU a day as a starting point, and more, as recommended by your health care provider, if you test deficient. Use this advice:

* **Ask your health care provider to test your blood levels of vitamin D to see if you are deficient.**

* **If you are deficient, ask your health care provider to monitor your blood as you take supplements.** This is the best way to find the best dose for you. For most of my patients, I recommend an average of 5,000 IU of vitamin D_3 daily until blood levels achieve 50 to 80 ng/dl. I reduce the dose if they exceed this range.

* **I recommend vitamin D_3, the form most commonly recommended.** It is usually derived from animal sources such as lanolin. If you are vegan and don't consume lanolin products, vegan versions of vitamin D_3 are now available.

Power Rx: Swallow Some Bacteria (Try Probiotics)

We harbor over three pounds of bacteria in our GI tract, mainly in the colon. A small number, less than 50 different species, are healthy and over 500 types may weaken our health.

Antibiotics, food additives, processed foods (excess fat, sugar, salt), excess alcohol, and food intolerances can alter the balance of bacteria in our gut. When the bad guys take hold, they produce harmful toxins that can leak into our bloodstreams. These toxins can irritate our blood vessels, setting the stage for heart disease. Research from the Cleveland Clinic has found that some harmful gut bacteria also turn lecithin—a nutrient in egg yolks, liver, beef, pork, and wheat germ—into an artery-clogging compound called trimethylamine-N-oxide (TMAO).[163]

Another a study presented at the 2012 American Heart Association Scientific Sessions found that twice daily doses of a probiotic supplement that contained *Lactobacillus reuteri* bacteria lowered levels of the bad LDL cholesterol by 11 percent over nine weeks. Total cholesterol dropped nine percent, too.[164]

Rx at a Glance

A probiotic supplement can tip the balance of your gut bacteria back to healthy by adding billions of disease-preventing microbes to your GI tract.

I recommend a probiotic to my patients. These are usually found in capsule form. Look for a supplement that contains at least 10 billion organisms and take it once daily. Also:

* **Eat fermented foods like sauerkraut, kimchi, and fermented vegetables.** These have billions of healthy probiotics in them and can be made easily at home.

* **Always take a probiotic whenever you are on any antibiotic.**

Power Rx: Take a Daily Aspirin

Technically an over-the-counter drug and not a supplement, aspirin is something I recommend daily for most of my patients with any variety of heart disease, even if it's just a slightly abnormal calcium score.

Aspirin interferes with the body's ability to clot. Usually, when you bleed, clotting cells (called platelets) in your blood go to the site of the wound and literally form a clog or plug in the hole, stopping the bleeding. This can happen inside the blood vessels, too, especially if the platelets are attempting to plug up injuries to the lining of your arteries. If blood clots form quickly, they can completely clog an artery, causing a heart attack.

Aspirin thins the blood and reduces the action of platelets, thus cutting your risk for sudden heart attack.

Still, it's not for everyone. You don't want to be on aspirin if you have a bleeding disorder. Also, some people are allergic to it.

Rx at a Glance

Use this advice to take the best dose of aspirin for you:

* **If you have never suffered a heart event, take 81 mg (the amount in one baby aspirin) a day.**

* **If you've had a heart attack or received a stent, talk to your health care provider about taking 325 mg,** which is the amount in a regular-strength tablet.

* **If you are about to have surgery—even dental surgery—tell your physician that you are taking aspirin.** You'll want to discuss whether you should stop taking it several days before to prevent bleeding complications.

* **If you are allergic to aspirin, consider other natural blood thinners** like nattokinase, ginkgo biloba, and even omega-3 fish oils.

Power Rx: Take Additional Supplements, as Needed

What follows is a list of the supplements that I commonly recommend for my heart patients, along with why I recommend them. Depending on your lifestyle, current state of health, diet, and other factors, they might be right for you, too:

L-carnitine. To produce ATP and power the heart, your mitochondria need fuel. Most of the fuel for your heart consists of fatty acids. There is a shuttle that helps fatty acids move across cell membranes to enter the energy pool. This shuttle requires L-carnitine to function at its peak. So taking oral L-carnitine either as a pill or as a powder can make more fatty acids available for energy production. Take 500 to 1,000 mg twice a day.

D-ribose. Another supplement that enhances mitochondrial energy production is a powder called D-ribose that looks and tastes like sugar. When studying the chemistry of the ATP molecule, Ohio cardiologist James Roberts, MD, observed that a key component of ATP is a ribose molecule. Ribose was already being used to treat fibromyalgia and boost exercise performance. Dr. Roberts and other cardiologists started adding D-ribose powder as a supplement for patients with heart failure and saw improvements in breathing, energy, and well-being. I have also used this strategy in hundreds of patients and can vouch for the boost in vitality. Aim for five grams, two to three times a day. Sprinkle ribose powder on blueberries or blackberries or add it to your smoothie for a tasty way to combine heart energy support with potent natural antioxidant foods.

Magnesium. Due to inadequate vegetable intake and depletion of the soil of building block nutrients, many people are deficient in magnesium. Furthermore, many heart patients are being treated with a diuretic, or water pill, that may rob the body of magnesium and worsen mitochondrial function. Supplementing with magnesium can lower blood pressure, normalize irregular beats, ease anxiety, enhance sleep, reduce headaches, resolve constipation, and most importantly, improve the energy level of heart patients and others. Tied with CoQ10, magnesium supplements may be the most frequent and beneficial addition I prescribe to my patients. The dosage is usually 250 to 500 mg a day. Use a chelated form like magnesium malate or magnesium glycinate. These are less likely to cause GI symptoms and I find they are especially helpful for patients with extra heartbeats and high blood pressure. Magnesium citrate is another good form. Avoid magnesium oxide, the most common form, because it is poorly absorbed. The one exception to this rule is when you are trying to whip constipation because this form of magnesium stays mainly in the GI tract.

B-complex vitamins. B vitamins support a key process called methylation, which regulates homocysteine levels and plays an important role in the control of DNA regulation. People with the MTHFR genetic inherited disorder may need special methylated B vitamins. The form I take, Vessel Care by Metagenics, has 800 µg of methylfolate, 1 mg of methylcobalamin, and 25 mg of vitamin B_6 as pyridoxine hydrochloride. Vitamin B_{12}, in particular, is especially important for vegetarians and vegans to take, because plants have less vitamin B_{12} than animal products. If you are vegetarian or vegan, you can either choose to take a B-complex vitamin (which will include B_{12}) or take vitamin B_{12} alone. In that case, I recommend taking 500 μg daily or 2,500 μg once a week, ideally as a liquid, sublingual, or chewable form for better absorption.

Taurine. Taurine is important to your cardiac health, immune system, insulin action, hearing, and electrolyte balance. Because it's typically found in meat and seafood, vegans and vegetarians often have low levels of taurine. Supplementation with 1,000 mg a day is a reasonable option, although doses of 1.5 to 3 mg a day are used in diabetic and cardiac patients. Energy drinks often contain taurine, but I don't recommend getting your taurine from these drinks due to their caffeine and sugar.

N-acetyl cysteine (NAC). This is a building block for glutathione, an antioxidant within your cells. It can help control blood pressure and may help ensure that patients taking nitroglycerin preparations by mouth or patch do not become tolerant to them, negating their impact. Take 600 mg a day.

Resveratrol. This polyphenol is found in grapes, peanuts, and famously, red wine. Associated with longevity in wine-loving communities like Sardinia, Italy, resveratrol is known to increase the activity of a family of genes called sirtuins that battle inflammation and oxidation and may be important at slowing aging. Take 250 mg of trans-resveratrol daily.

Alpha-lipoic acid. This powerful antioxidant has been shown to halt or reverse diabetic peripheral neuropathy. It may protect mitochondria from oxidative damage. Take 300 mg a day. A form of ALA called R-lipoic acid is more potent.

L-theanine. This green tea extract provides a calming effect without sedation, may enhance sleep, and lowers blood pressure. It has proven very safe in my practice in patients with high stress and anxiety levels. Take 200 mg twice a day.

Ashwagandha: This Indian herb is also very useful for patients struggling with stress and anxiety. I find 400 to 500 mg twice a day provides results.

Berberine: Derived from plants, berberine has been shown to lower blood sugar and cholesterol levels. It has been found in small studies to improve heart function, but further research is needed. I usually recommend 500 mg once or twice a day.

Green tea extracts concentrating EGCG (epigallocatechin gallate): These are useful for cholesterol and triglyceride control, antioxidant activity, and reducing arterial stiffness in patients with congestive heart failure. EGCG at 500 mg twice a day has resulted in good responses in my patients.

Rx at a Glance

Supplements and prescription medicines sometimes interact in strange ways. For instance, certain supplements (and even some foods) can block or increase the absorption of certain medicines. Certain medicines can also block the absorption of certain nutrients. And some supplements are capable of interacting with each other. This is where a good relationship with your health care provider and pharmacist will come in handy. This is what I recommend you do:

* **Bring this book with you to your next appointment.** If that feels like too much, then, at the very least, copy the chart on page 265 and bring that. Talk about the pros and cons of various supplements and ask your health care provider what he or she recommends.

* **Write down which supplements and medicines you take.** Take note of the dosage, how many times a day you take each, and the brand. Make sure your health care provider is aware of this. Bring your list to your health care provider or pharmacist and ask if any of

them might interact. If so, ask him or her to suggest alternatives.

* **Copy the chart below and take it to your health care provider.** Use this handy resource to guide your discussion about which supplements are right for you.

	Vegan	Existing Heart Disease	On Diuretics	On Statins	High Blood Pressure	High Cholesterol
Multivitamin	X	X	X	X	X	X
Vitamin D	X	X	X	X	X	X
Probiotics	X	X	X	X	X	X
CoQ10	X	X	X	X	X	X
Selenium		X				
L-carnitine	X	X			X	X
D-ribose		X				
Magnesium		X	X		X	
B-complex	X	X				
Taurine	X				X	
Aspirin		X			X	
N-acetyl cysteine		X			X	
Resveratrol					X	X
Alpha-lipoic acid		X			X	
L-theanine					X	
Ashwagandha					X	
Berberine		X			X	X
Green tea extracts		X				X

YOUR FINAL SUPPLEMENT RX

That's a lot. I know. It's probably overwhelming. For most patients, I suggest a base supplement program that includes vitamin D_3 if their blood level is low, a probiotic, CoQ10, and antioxidants usually found in a natural plant-based multivitamin. That's it.

Some, of course, depending on their health concerns, take a lot more. No matter how few or how many supplements you take, it bears repeating: Your pills are never a substitute for real food. Rather, they are an adjunct to a healthy diet. Pair them with plant-based whole foods featuring many leafy green vegetables, beans, raw nuts, and seeds.

Chapter 12

Your Plan for a Lasting Heart

Albert Einstein is credited with saying, "The definition of insanity is doing the same thing over and over again and expecting different results."

You picked up this book for a reason. Maybe you had a health scare. Maybe one of your high school buddies walked into a bank last week, filled out a deposit slip, and then, before he ever got to the teller, dropped dead from a sudden heart attack . . . one he never saw coming. You thought, "That could have been me."

Maybe you just learned that your cholesterol or blood pressure is too high.

Or perhaps there was another reason.

No matter the reason, you now know how to prevent the world's number one killer from claiming your life. So the question is this: Will you become a living, breathing example of Einstein's definition of insanity? Will you continue to do the same things, eat the same foods, and practice the same lifestyle habits, but expect a different result?

Or will you do something different?

It's my hope that you choose sanity.

In Chapters 6 through 11, I gave you dozens of prescriptions. For easy reference, you'll find a list of them here.

Nutrition Prescriptions

* Eat leafy greens to lower blood pressure all day long.
* Add spices to everything.
* Buy organic.
* Drink more tea.
* Break up with soda and other sweetened beverages.
* Enjoy coffee in moderation.
* Eat more plants (at least five servings a day).
* Study food labels like Jane Goodall studies chimps.
* Skip foods made in plants.
* Drive past the drive-thru.
* If you eat meat, avoid hormones and antibiotics.
* If you eat meat, consume it only after dark.
* Swap SMASH fish in for meat.
* Temporarily take a break from dairy and wheat.
* Go vegan.

Food Prep Prescriptions

* Do a clean sweep of your kitchen.
* Shop along the edges of the grocery store.
* Break the record for the person who eats the slowest.
* Tune in to the pleasure of eating.
* Do your own food prep.

* Avoid heart AGErs with smart cooking techniques.
* Drink your veggies.
* Chew your fruit (avoid fruit juice).
* Cook once, eat five times.
* Fast 11 hours every night.

Fitness Prescriptions

* Take a five-minute walk.
* Never fast-forward through a commercial.
* Practice active acts of kindness.
* De-motorvate your life.
* Don't take waiting sitting down.
* Get a pedometer.
* Stand whenever possible.
* If you miss a week, don't throw in the towel.
* Take vitamin Y (try yoga).
* Move in the morning.
* Invest $10 a month in movement.
* Stay out of your comfort zone.
* Go hard for 20 seconds.
* Walk while you work.
* Run long distances like a turtle.

Emotional Health Prescriptions

* Laugh at least once a day.
* Drop blood pressure in five minutes by counting your breaths.
* Breathe through one side of your nose.

* Breathe out the tension.
* Count your blessings.
* Meditate your stress away.
* Meditate your anger away, too.
* Cuddle with a pet.
* Get busy.
* Sleep seven to eight hours at night.
* Walk in the sun for 15 minutes.
* Embrace volunteer work.
* Take vitamin Y (try yoga).
* Try tai chi.
* Get a little breathing help from your apps.
* Join a group of like-minded people.
* Try waon therapy.
* Try acupuncture.
* Ground yourself.

Eco Prescriptions

* Open your windows to reduce indoor air pollution.
* If you exercise outdoors, do it in the morning.
* If you live in a city, wear noise-cancelling headphones.
* Avoid smoke.
* Don't drink petroleum (ditch plastic water bottles).
* Make your kitchen a plastic-free zone.
* Don't put anything on your skin that you wouldn't eat.
* Study ingredient labels like Jane Goodall studies chimps.

* Clean with food, not with chemicals.
* Air out your dry cleaning.
* Keep your phone at arm's length.

Supplement Prescriptions

* Do a background check on your supplements.
* Take natural multivitamins.
* Buy supplements from trusted sources.
* Take Coenzyme Q10 (CoQ10).
* Try this pill of sunshine (vitamin D).
* Swallow some bacteria (try probiotics).
* Take a daily aspirin.
* Take additional supplements, as needed.

Take a close look. What strategies have you already incorporated into your life? Which ones could you incorporate easily, perhaps as soon as today or tomorrow? Which ones do you think you could tackle within a few weeks? A few months? A year?

Make a promise to yourself right now, and make that promise very real. Buy yourself a journal. Let's call it your Lasting Heart Log. Decorate it if you want. Draw or paste inspiring pictures such as your dream of how you one day want to look and feel, memories of active days you spent with your grandkids—days you hope will continue, or something that reminds you of a happy time, such as photos of your wedding or anniversary. Or leave it plain. That's up to you. It doesn't have to be fancy. It only needs to be something you use.

On the first page of the journal, write today's date and the word "Before."

On the line just under that, write down everything you already know about your current state of health. This is where you might want to take note of your weight, cholesterol reading, blood pressure, and blood sugar. It's also where you want to jot down your calcium score and results of other tests that I recommend in Chapter 4.

Then, fill the rest of the page with the current state of your lifestyle, and be honest. Based on what you learned in *The Whole Heart Solution*, what are you doing everyday that speeds premature aging of your heart and blood vessels? Conversely, what are you not doing everyday that could be slowing their demise?

What do you usually eat for breakfast? Lunch? Dinner? And snacks? What beverages do you consume throughout the day? Write it all down.

* Do you smoke? Make a note of how many packs a day.

* How about exercise? What are you currently doing?

* How much television do you watch? How much time do you spend in front of a computer or tablet?

* What's your current level of stress? Rate it on a 1 to 10 scale.

* How long is your commute?

* How many servings of fruits and vegetables are you getting in a given day?

* What types of relaxation strategies are you using? What types do you wish you were using?

* How many toxic products do you use?

* How many meat-, dairy-, and egg-free meals do you consume a week?

* Number of fried meals a week?

* Number of doughnuts or processed carbohydrates a week?

* How about fast food?

* Purchases of organic produce?

* Products purchased without trans fats?

* Products purchased without high fructose corn syrup and GMO sources?

* Number of artificial sweeteners and sugar-sweetened beverages?

* Glasses of spring or filtered water consumed?

* Tea?

* Percentage of your food budget spent on the outside perimeter of the store?

* Number of hours slept?

* How many times do you laugh each day?

* Type of supplements used?

Write down as much as you can think of, even if it all spans more than a page. Once you've finished, draw a big, thick, symbolic line. That's your line where the unhealthy heart habits stop and the healthier habits start.

On the next page, write "After." As you change your lifestyle, write down every single success, no matter how seemingly minor. If you buy organic apples for the first time, write it down.

The day you consume one more vegetable serving than the day before: Get out the notebook.

It's the same every time you replace a toxic household product with a non-toxic one. If you buy a bottle of vitamin D, make a note of it.

What follows are several key moments my patients have shared with me from their Lasting Heart Logs:

* "Parked in the space farthest from the building. It actually made me smile when I waved someone else into the close space I usually claim for myself."

* "Tried kale. Wasn't as bad as I thought. Actually, I kinda liked it."

* "Asked the waiter to leave the cheese off the burrito."

* "Got a massage!"

* "Asked if I could work from home so I can walk around the neighborhood during the hour I'm usually in my car."

* "Did my first meatless meal."

* "Bought that NutriBullet blender Dr. Kahn keeps telling me about."

* "Tried a green smoothie. It sure didn't taste how it looked!"

* "Got to an appointment early. Walked around the building while I waited."

* "Watched the DVD *Forks Over Knives* and went a week without meat."

* "Tore up my last pack of cigarettes and am using patches."

* "Went to a vegetarian restaurant and had a stir-fry, yum."

* "Made juice for the first time at home and survived."

This record keeping might seem tedious, but it can be very helpful. In my experience of caring for patients for over 20 years, and in my own life, change comes gradually, so gradually that many of us don't even realize we are changing at all. We move forward slowly, one step at a time.

ALL ROADS LEAD TO HOLISTIC HEALTH

How quickly you change your eating, moving, thinking, and supplement habits will probably depend, in large part, on your current state of health and the skills and knowledge you have to make the changes. By the time patients come to see me, they are often very motivated. That's usually because they've experienced chest pain or some other symptom, had a procedure, or they were prescribed a medicine they wished they didn't have to take. They thought, "I don't want to be sick." And they decided to do everything they could to reverse their poor health, reduce the need for meds, and extend their number of years on the planet. Usually they still need some coaching in specific steps to take, hence *The Whole Heart Solution.*

An example of one of these super-motivated people was Ted, a patient who came to see me after he'd survived a heart attack. It literally scared him almost to death and he wanted better for himself and his family. He read every book and watched every video I recommended and bought appliances for his kitchen to make the trip easier. He emptied out his pantry and freezer of old "heart attack foods," and I guided him in buying foods from an entirely new grocery list. His journey to a healthy, lasting heart was swift and effective. During the first six weeks, this is what he focused on during a typical day.

* **5:30 a.m.** He wakes refreshed because, after committing to sleeping seven hours most nights, he went to bed at 10:30 p.m. the night before rather than watch a late-night movie.

* **5:45 a.m.** On Mondays and Fridays he commits to listening to a relaxing tape that teaches him to meditate.

* **6:15 a.m.** Every other day he does 30 minutes of cardio, weights, and stretching.

* **6:45 a.m.** He grabs a greens and berry smoothie with a protein powder and flax seeds.

* **7:15 a.m.** He leaves for work with a packed lunch and snacks of raw nuts, an apple, and a hummus and tabbouleh wrap.

* **8 a.m.–noon** He takes breaks at least once an hour to stand, pace, and stretch.

* **Noon** He has lunch, which on a typical day might be a huge salad packed with greens, nuts, avocados, and strips of tempeh (an easy option because he can slice the tempeh as soon as he pulls it from the package).

* **Noon–5 p.m.** He takes breaks at least once an hour to stand, pace, and stretch.

* **Early evening** He has a home-cooked meal, which might be a stir-fry of vegetables and beans on a bed of brown rice. He drinks one glass of pinot noir with dinner. If he's still hungry, he snacks on raw carrots and celery.

Ted is my hero, because that's quite a bit of change to accomplish in only six weeks. But remember: He was a heart attack survivor. You might say Ted was extremely motivated, because he was. But the point is that this is a progression. Ted didn't try every single prescription at once. He even broke down some prescriptions into smaller goals. For instance, notice that he didn't just start meditating every day. He started by listening to a tape twice a week.

Let's take a look at Ted's typical day about four months later.

* **5:45 a.m.** Ted meditates daily for 20 minutes.

* **6:15 a.m.** On days he is not doing cardio and weights, Ted follows a yoga teaching series on DVD.

* **6:45 a.m.** Ted uses the juicer he purchased and the produce he stocks in his fridge to make a juice filled with a variety of organic vegetables and fruits. Three

times a week one of these is a green juice infused with lemon, ginger, cayenne pepper, and turmeric. He has a more substantial snack later in the morning of fruit and an open-faced tofu sandwich on gluten-free toast.

* **Noon** At work, Ted started a walking group. They meet at lunch and walk briskly for 20 minutes. He has found that the conversation and support are as much benefit as the movement. Then he still has a few minutes to eat the lunch he packed for himself of a brown rice vegetable dish that he made in bulk earlier in the week.

* **Early evening** Ted now grows sprouts and has added living foods to his diet in salads and juices. He starts dinner with a huge salad topped with these sprouts, and then follows up with vegetable-quinoa casserole or some other homemade delight.

* **10:30 p.m.** It is bedtime. Ted reviews his day and is grateful for many things, including the good choices he made to promote his health. He goes to sleep on his grounding sheets.

I hope you agree with me that Ted is doing great, and no matter where you are four months into your journey, you are doing great, too. Just try to do more than you were doing before. That's what's most important.

Now let's take a look at where Ted was a year into this new lifestyle.

* **5:45–6:45 a.m.** Ted continues the meditation and exercise routines, followed by his healthy breakfast of fruit and oatmeal.

* **7 a.m.** Ted has replaced his toothpaste, soaps, shampoos, and deodorants with toxin-free versions he has read about at www.ewg.org.

* **During the workday** Ted continues to walk during any breaks and meet his walking group. He also continues to pack his lunch and snacks.

* **5 p.m.** On his way home from work, Ted picks up the dry cleaning from an eco-friendly company he has researched. As soon as he gets home, he takes it out of the plastic and hangs it in the garage for a day to de-gas.

* **5:30 p.m.** Ted has found a wellness center that offers a half hour of infrared sauna therapy for $20. He enjoys the detoxifying, sweaty experience.

* **Early evening** Ted has a healthy, home-cooked dinner of vegetable bean soup (made in his slow cooker while he was at work) with a side of baked potato.

Now for the best part. During the year he was making lifestyle changes, Ted's body was responding with changes of its own. He lost 14 pounds, slashed his blood pressure and cholesterol, lowered his calcium score, and now feels energetic and light.

I'm thrilled for him.

Of course, not everyone is as motivated as Ted. I like to think of him as my star student. Other patients incorporate prescriptions into their lives more slowly. If Ted's progression sounds intense and too swift for you, then you might be more like Carol. She still felt great, had no symptoms of heart disease, and probably would not have changed a thing had not a routine cholesterol test revealed that she had abnormally high levels of the dangerous small, dense LDL cholesterol. When she came to see me, she had one goal: avoid taking the cholesterol-lowering medication that her health care provider had strongly advised she start right away. I told her that her diet was the best place to start. Even small dietary changes could add up to big results. After talking with Carol, I learned that her diet consisted mainly of three food groups: diet soft drinks, processed convenience foods, and meat.

She consumed one or two servings of produce a day, usually in the form of a processed potato product or ketchup. She was always in a rush and grabbed convenient, but deadly, foods.

Carol decided to start by improving her P/A (plant to animal) ratio, and she focused on making over breakfast first. She read an article I had written called "Is Your Breakfast Killing You?" and she was impressed. Rather than grabbing an egg sandwich on her way to work, she began stopping off at a nearby smoothie business instead. At first, she ordered the strawberry and banana smoothie, which allowed her to start her day with two servings of fruit. Over time, she became more and more adventurous. One day she decided to try the "green" smoothie, a drink that was loaded mostly with fruit, but that also contained spinach. She raved about the drink, and just could not believe how good something so green could possibly taste.

From there, she took the big step of buying a blender and making her own smoothies at home. This allowed her to use more vegetables and less sugar and fruit, increasing her P/A ratio even more.

With breakfast under control, she moved on to snacks—most of which, initially, were chips and desserts that she ate on impulse. I suggested that she plan her snacks ahead of time. That way she'd be less likely to fall prey to temptation. So, once a week, Carol stocked up on plant-based, whole food snacks such as apples, oranges, grapes, celery sticks, carrot sticks, and raw nuts and seeds.

Now it was time to move on to lunch. Carol usually ate this meal in the company cafeteria, so her first step was a simple one: vegetablize anything she typically ordered. She began topping every burger, sandwich, and wrap with an assortment of veggies. That first step proved easy for her, so she then began adding a vegetable side dish from the salad bar. After that, she made it her goal to pack lunch once a week. Soon she was up to two, and then three days a week. Before long, she was packing most days.

From there, she moved on to dinner. For this meal, Carol invested in a few cookbooks, especially one that featured slow cooker recipes. She assembled the meals in the morning, and they were ready for her by the time she arrived home from work.

With just those changes alone, Carol's blood cholesterol improved dramatically, and so did her overall energy. She felt so good that she decided to incorporate more and more whole heart prescriptions, even though she'd already met her health goal.

As you can see, Carol and Ted tackled their whole heart prescriptions very differently, and this is true of every patient I've counseled. Some start with prescriptions from Chapter 10 because they feel it's easier to simply buy different brands of the products they use every day. Others start with the emotional health prescriptions, mostly because, in addition to poor heart health, they also want to overcome their negativity and stress.

Others start with food because they want to make the most effective changes first.

Some start simply by watching a video or by buying a new appliance.

You might want to start somewhere else.

The point is that you start with something, no matter how small a change it might seem to you. Maybe you decide, for instance, to read one label of one product in your kitchen. Or maybe instead of a double cheeseburger, you have a hamburger with just one patty.

Or maybe you decide to stop at that smoothie place at the mall and see what they have to offer.

It doesn't matter how small a goal you set for yourself as long as you set one, and then keep moving in the right direction.

Your Lasting Heart Log will help you notice all the steps you take in the right direction, giving you a clear picture of just how far you've come. You might think that you can just take note of your progress in your head. I've found, however, that many people quickly forget their progress. Instead, they focus on how much they haven't yet accomplished. And by fixating on their failures, they demotivate themselves all the way back to zero.

That's why I recommend you read over your Lasting Heart Log

once a week. As you do so, smile about all you've done. At the beginning of each week, you might even jot down some goals for the week to come. At the end of the week, check and see if you got it all done.

Then, twice a year, reassess your health. Write in a new weight. If you undergo new tests, jot down your results. Compare them to the year before.

Also, look at the big picture. Look over the notes you've taken in the past year and compare them to your "Before" page. Do a little math. What's the number of personal care, household, and garage products that you've converted to non-toxic and environmentally friendly? How many times do you now laugh in a day? Minutes spent breathing deeply? Time spent volunteering? Moments spent walking barefoot? Time in an infrared sauna?

If you didn't change as much for the better as you would have liked, then use that as motivation to fully incorporate more prescriptions. Reread sections of the book for inspiration or whenever you feel stuck. Add new habits slowly.

Over time, as you add more habits, something amazing will happen. You'll feel better. Remember: It takes an entire body to beat a heart. That means everything that strengthens your heart also strengthens every cell in your body. As your heart grows younger, so does every other part of you. Soon you'll have more energy. You'll also be in a better mood. You'll feel less stress. And things that once felt hard—such as having the stamina to play tag with the grandkids—will feel easy.

That's your greatest reward. Use that newfound Fountain of Youth as inspiration to incorporate more and more prescriptions into your life.

In this way you will build a lasting heart, one change at a time. I wish you much success. May the beat go on!

Resources

Please think of this book as the beginning of your heart education and not the end.

Long ago I was told that the books you read and the people you meet will change your life. Now that has to be broadened to include websites, documentaries, and webinars. I regularly read books on health promotion. Lectures and festivals dedicated to healthy living options are more frequent than ever. I urge you to also develop a habit of reading or watching at least several health programs a year, as well as scanning the print or digital media to learn of new developments. To help you reach that goal, I am listing some of the resources that I find most helpful.

WEBSITES

PubMed.com. This free database is maintained by the National Library of Medicine. It contains more than 22 million references on medicine. Many references go back well over 50 years, and about 500,000 new citations are added yearly. These are scientific medical articles from print and electronic journals. Many are peer-reviewed journals, which means that the article must be reviewed and often corrected before it is accepted for publication. PubMed is where I go to research medical topics. For example, when I enter the terms "sauna" and "congestive heart failure" in the search area, 51 medical references show up. Many, but not all, give access to the full article, and for the majority of the rest at least a paragraph abstract is available. It is interesting to find out how much actual science is behind a "hot topic" on the Internet. For example, I have been interested in the potential advantages of natural vitamins from plant-based sources versus synthetic vitamins that are often cheaper but can be made even from petrochemicals. On a search engine like Google or Bing, this topic will bring up dozens of websites generally favoring the natural vitamin sources for your health. On PubMed, there are surprisingly few research articles on the topic, and those that exist are mainly in horses and pigs!

Danielplan.com. I mentioned the Daniel Plan in Chapter 8. If you remember, Saddleback Church initiated a faith-based wellness effort for their massive congregation a few years ago. They brought in Drs. Mark Hyman, Daniel Amen, and Mehmet Oz to design and lead a small group and web-based lifestyle change effort. The program drew 16,000 participants in the first week and has grown internationally. I brought this plan to my synagogue along with another doctor and supportive rabbis. We substituted some different Bible teachings, but the core medical information is fantastic. There are articles, videos, blogs, and frequent updates. I strongly urge you to spend some time on the many pages of this site.

pcrm.org. The Physicians Committee for Responsible Medicine or PCRM is a nearly 30-year-old organization founded by Dr. Neal Barnard to advocate for nutrition guidelines, healthy school programs, and animal rights, amongst other topics. Dr. Barnard has authored many books and blogs, which are posted regularly. PCRM has a wonderful 21-day Kickstart program to explore a plant-based diet. Recipes and encouragement arrive by email if you sign up for this free lifestyle change program.

peta.org. This well-known organization, People for the Ethical Treatment of Animals, advocates vocally for animal rights. It is also a website packed with plans and suggestions for lifestyle changes, including hundreds of vegetarian recipes. A simple program to sample a vegetarian lifestyle is available for free, including a three-week starter program.

nutritionfacts.org. Dr. Michael Greger launched this free website several years ago and now creates daily short videos examining some aspect of plant-based nutrition. Dr. Greger has a sharp eye for interesting topics and a keen sense of humor that make watching these short courses enjoyable. I look forward to the daily arrival of his emails and have learned what is the tea with the highest antioxidant level, what is the vegetable with the highest arginine content for arteries, how red and white wine compare in inhibiting the aromatase enzyme, and so on. I would make it a part of your daily routine.

mercola.com. Few Internet figures in the medical sphere are as controversial as Dr. Joseph Mercola, but his daily updates have become a staple of my reading. I am often at odds with his recommendations, but his dedication to promoting the eating of an organic, non-GMO, and vegetable-rich diet is constant.

drfuhrman.com. Dr. Joel Fuhrman is a successful author and is often seen on PBS. His website has many searchable features on nutrition and vitamin supplements.

lef.org. Life Extension Foundation has been manufacturing high-quality vitamin supplements for several decades and their website is rich in resource materials on vitamins and nutrition. They were amongst the first to recommend CoQ10, vitamin D, and fish oil as routine supplements, and they have a board of advisors made up of well-respected scientists and physicians. Their monthly publication, *Life Extension Magazine*, can be ordered for free for the first three months and has fascinating articles that are heavily referenced from the medical literature.

mindbodygreen.com. This relatively new website has guest bloggers who post articles on yoga, wellness, nutrition, and health. It is now read by millions of people each month. I have contributed many articles on cardiovascular health, and you can search my name to read them. But don't just read my articles! The site also offers an Internet-based training course on how to eat a plant-based diet, how to meditate, and how to practice yoga. The quality and value of these teaching modules are exceptional. I highly recommend them.

sciencedaily.com. This website is packed with articles on all kinds of scientific topics. A button on Health and Medicine draws you to topics on the human body and another button takes you to topics on heart disease. I often find the articles interesting, well referenced, and helpful for following the rapid advances that are occurring.

oldwayspt.org. This website is based in Boston and is a wealth of information on the Mediterranean diet. The nonprofit organization Old Ways was the first to publish a Mediterranean food pyramid in 1993. There are scientific references, recipes, and charts. There are vegetarian, African American, Latino, and Asian versions of the Mediterranean diet. This site is worth searching and sharing with others.

vsh.org. The Vegetarian Society of Hawaii seems to have no problem getting world leaders on healthy eating and environmental issues to travel to Hawaii and lecture on interesting topics. I wonder why? The lectures are fascinating and are posted for viewing for free on this site, with a new one each month.

vegsource.com. This colorful website has many articles, recipes, eating plans, and shopping options that make a vegetarian lifestyle easy. There are also links to over 50 other websites that are full of useful information.

ewg.org. The Environmental Working Group has been mentioned several times in this book and is a resource that everyone can benefit from. The sections on safe choices for consumer products, household cleaning items, sunscreens, and non-GMO foods are a must-read. The Dirty Dozen list of produce, such as apples and celery, is an important guide to intelligent shopping.

ted.com. This Internet sensation includes short lectures given by some of the most brilliant experts, or 1,000 "ideas worth sharing." I will often search the site for medical talks, and I am never disappointed.

VIDEOS

Forks Over Knives. This 2011 film has its own website, www.forksoverknives.com, and has led to a number of DVDs and books. The film pays homage to two of my personal heroes, Dr. Caldwell Esselstyn of the Cleveland Clinic and Dr. T. Colin Campbell of Cornell University. Both men began life on meat farms but over the course of their medical and research careers, respectively, took a stance that plant-based diets were the optimal way to eat to prevent and reverse disease. The movie also looks at factory farming and its cruelty. I have found that this film changes people's view of eating animal products more than any other teaching tool.

Food, Inc. This 2008 documentary looks at the corporate farming of animals and displays the dark side of about 75 million animals a day—in the United States alone—being slaughtered for food production. Confined animal factory organizations (CAFO) are a development of only the last few decades, and the movie demonstrates why current legislation in some states makes it a crime to film the poor conditions of the big food manufacturers. Well worth the time.

Super Size Me. This 2004 classic describes the 30-day mission of Morgan Spurlock to eat at nothing but McDonald's restaurants. The changes in his weight, cholesterol, and blood sugar are enough to ensure that you steer far past a fast food restaurant for the good of your health.

Fat, Sick and Nearly Dead. This is a 2010 documentary about Joe Cross, an overweight Australian man with many pills and health issues. He arrives in New York and travels across the United States with a juicer and vegetables, drinking his Mean

Green Juice, exclusively, for two months. In the process he loses over 80 pounds and meets many other people struggling with their weight and health. Joe gets off his medications and stops suffering from many years of an autoimmune condition requiring steroid therapy. The website www.fatsickandnearlydead.com is very helpful when you begin to juice. I found this movie so compelling that I bought my first juicer and started to use it regularly right after viewing it. Thanks, Joe. I attended one of his lectures recently, and he is dynamic, articulate, and passionate about juicing, even with whole foods, to add an easy source of vitamins and nutrients to our cells.

Simply Raw. There are two long-established centers in the United States that teach a lifestyle featuring living, raw, organic, and sprouted foods. One is the Hippocrates Health Institute in West Palm Beach, Florida, and the other is the Tree of Life Center in Patagonia, Arizona. The latter center is led by Dr. Gabriel Cousens, a Columbia University–trained physician. The documentary *Simply Raw* (2011) demonstrates six examples of how just 30 days of changing eating habits can get most adult diabetics off medications. I have great respect for Dr. Cousens. The burden that diabetes is placing on adults throughout the world is tremendous. If you are frustrated with taking too many pills or injections, this documentary will be of interest to you.

HEALTH AND WELLNESS AUTHORS

John Robbins. In 1987, John Robbins wrote the book *Diet for a New America*, which laid out the argument that for medical, environmental, and animal cruelty reasons, plant-based eating was the best choice. In that same year, someone handed me a copy of this book as I was boarding a plane for a few days of hiking in Aspen with my wife, Karen. I was a fellow in training in cardiology and the clarity of the message in the book was so strong that we both became committed vegetarians that trip (we were pretty close already but did not understand the full basis for a green lifestyle). Robbins is interesting in that his father was the founder of the Baskin-Robbins ice cream chain, but he rejected the offer of working in the family business and moved to British Columbia to live a simple life with his young wife and son. Subsequent books by Robbins such as *Food Revolution* and *Healthy at 100* continue to educate the public about the reasons for shunning animal products in favor of plant-based living.

Nathan Pritikin. Nathan Pritikin passed away in 1985. He wrote several books including the *Pritikin Program for Diet and Exercise*. Since his passing, his legacy has been maintained. In 2008, cardiologist Robert Vogel, MD, wrote *The Pritikin Edge, 10 Essential Ingredients for a Long and Delicious Life*. The book outlines the program that Pritikin developed to prevent and reverse heart disease that is now certified by the U.S. reimbursement community as a Pritikin Intensive Cardiac Rehabilitation program.

Dean Ornish, MD. Dr. Dean Ornish, a California cardiologist, challenged the established cardiac community when he began treating patients with advanced heart disease with low-fat, plant-based diets, exercise, smoking cessation, and stress management, leading to stunning results in the Lifestyle Heart Trial. His book, *Dr. Dean Ornish's Program for Reversing Heart Disease*, first published in 1990, continues to be a classic well worth reading. His subsequent works, such as *The Spectrum* (published in 2008), are groundbreaking in that they combine scientific outcomes with lifestyle changes.

Neal Barnard, MD. Dr. Neal Barnard, director and founder of the Physician's Committee for Responsible Medicine (www.pcrm. org), has authored 12 books since 1990; his most recent one is *Power Foods for the Brain*. His earlier book, *Dr. Neal Barnard's Program for Reversing Diabetes*, was based on clinical research he headed up that was published in peer-reviewed medical journals. Dr. Barnard is also a great lecturer and can be found on PBS and social media websites such as www.ted.com.

Caldwell Esselstyn, MD. This senior surgeon at the Cleveland Clinic starting gathering cardiac patients with advanced heart disease in the 1980s and placing them on plant-based, low-fat diets. He followed them and had repeat stress tests and catheterizations in many of them, showing reversal of disease with diet alone. He is featured in the documentary *Forks Over Knives* and his book *Prevent and Reverse Heart Disease* is not to be missed. I have sent patients to spend a day with Dr. Esselstyn and his wonderful wife Ann to be immersed in plant-based food preparation. I have also had the privilege of lecturing with Dr. Esselstyn, and he is a force.

Joel Fuhrman, MD. This family physician is a successful author and educator on the healing power of plant-based diets. He stresses evaluating the nutritional value of food and has developed a scoring system for the Whole Foods grocery chain, the ANDI scoring system. His books, *Eat to Live* and *Eat for Health*, were *New York Times* bestsellers. I have recommended his books to many patients and they have made substantial changes following the program.

Colin T. Campbell, MD. This professor emeritus of nutritional biochemistry at Cornell University was featured in the movie *Forks Over Knives*. His book, *The China Study*, describes decades of research he performed on the connection between animal products—particularly the milk protein casein—and disease. He advocates low-fat, plant-based diets. The China Study is a must-read if you want to understand why you should change your diet. His second book, *Whole*, argues for whole food, plant-based diets as the foundation of disease prevention.

Gabriel Cousens, MD. Cousens founded the Tree of Life Center and has authored many books. His book *There Is a Cure for Diabetes* is an excellent resource for reversing blood sugar issues. *Spiritual Nutrition*, another classic, describes the connection between the mind and body in terms of diet.

Brian Clement, PhD, and Anna Maria Clement, PhD. This husband-and-wife team has written many books on nutrition and healthful lifestyles. *Living Foods for Optimum Health* is an excellent discourse on why eating raw, sprouted, and living foods enhances your health, and *Killer Clothes* is a fascinating read about the toxins in many articles of clothing.

Daniel Amen, MD. A well-known adult and child psychiatrist with a series of clinics emphasizing brain nuclear (SPECT) imaging to tailor treatment, Dr. Amen uses many herbal and vitamin preparations. He is the author of the 1999 *New York Times* bestseller *Change Your Brain, Change Your Life*. His book *The Amen Solution* offers a brain perspective.

Tana Amen, RN, BSB. Dr. Amen's wife, Tana, published *The OmniDiet*, which is an eating plan emphasizing 70 percent plant and 30 percent protein sources. This book also reached the *New York Times* bestseller list and prompted a PBS special. I have recommended it to many patients with great feedback.

Mark Hyman, MD. Dr. Hyman has dedicated his family practice career to understanding the root causes of disease and has written many excellent books. *The Blood Sugar Solution* addresses stabilizing blood sugar swings through frequent small meals and snacks using food as a medicine. He was instrumental in designing the Daniel Plan at Saddleback Church. He is a frequent lecturer and can be found on www.ted.com.

Stephen Sinatra, MD. A senior cardiologist in Connecticut, Dr. Sinatra has written many books. *Reverse Heart Disease Now* is an excellent manual for preventing heart disease. He is also the co-author of *Earthing with Clinton Ober*, the definitive book on grounding.

Jon Kabat-Zinn, PhD. Dr. Kabat-Zinn founded a type of meditation, used in many hospitals and clinics, known as mindfulness-based stress reduction. His book *Mindfulness for Beginners* is an excellent introduction.

Mark Houston, MD. A noted world expert on natural therapies of heart disease, Dr. Houston has written a number of books. His book *What Your Doctor May Not Tell You about Heart Disease* is not to be missed.

CENTERS FOR LIFESTYLE CHANGE

If you have the resources and drive, traveling to a center specializing in lifestyle change can be transforming. Several centers have distinguished themselves for offering programs that can last from one to three weeks and might just be the ticket you were looking for.

Pritikin Longevity Center and Spa (www.pritikin.com) is in Miami, Florida, and is based on the life and work of health pioneer Nathan Pritikin. This center is one of two lifestyle programs in the United States that has sufficient long-term follow-up of attendees from Intensive Cardiac Rehabilitation programs. As a result, insurance coverage is available for some candidates. Programs for heart health as short as one to two days are available.

Tree of Life Rejuvenation Center (www.treeoflife.nu) is in Patagonia, Arizona, about an hour from Tucson. There are also programs run in Israel. This center is led by Dr. Gabriel Cousens and offers programs of various lengths. There are facilities to stay at and medical testing and examinations are available. I have not visited this center but know many who have and the applause is deafening.

Hippocrates Health Institute (www.hippocratesinst.org) is in West Palm Beach, Florida, situated on 40 plush acres. The institute has a history dating back to the 1950s, when Ann Wigmore, the mother of wheatgrass and juicing, opened a facility in Boston. This later moved to Florida and has expanded under the guidance of husband and wife PhDs Brian and Anna Maria Clement. Life transformation programs are offered that generally last three weeks. The plan features organic, raw, and living foods including green juice drinks and wheatgrass. There may be up to 100 residents from around the world seeking healing from a variety of disorders. I have visited this center and it is a beautiful oasis of mind and body treatments and rejuvenation.

Dr. McDougall's Health and Medical Center (www.drmcdougall. com) is in Santa Rosa, California, and led by Dr. John McDougall.

Dr. McDougall has been a leader and prolific author for 40 years and lectures widely. He uses low-fat, plant-based foods to prevent and reverse diseases and has programs where you can live at the center for three to ten days. There are also trips offering the lifestyle change program in exotic sites like Costa Rica. Dr. McDougall has also developed programs for employees of corporations and companies like Whole Foods to send hundreds of higher-risk employees to the center to learn healthier living.

Canyon Ranch (www.canyonranch.com) is in both Tucson, Arizona, and Lenox, Massachusetts, but also has spa clubs in other locations. The two main campuses offer a week-long life enhancement program that has been serving clients for over 25 years. The program is medically supervised and surrounded by beautiful facilities.

Blum Center for Health (www.blumcenterforhealth.com) is located in Rye Brook, New York, and features three- to five-day immersions in healthy living and weight loss. The program is supervised by Dr. Susan Blum.

True North Health Center (www.healthpromoting.com) is in Santa Rosa, California, and offers 24 rooms and one of the most prestigious staffs of doctors and healers. They emphasize plant-based nutrition and fasting.

Endnotes

1. World Health Organization, "Global Status Report on Noncommunicable Diseases 2010," www.who.int/nmh/publications/ncd_report_full_en.

2. A. J. Epstein et al., "Coronary Revascularization Trends in the United States, 2001–2008," *Journal of the American Medical Association* 305, no. 17 (May 2011): 1769–76.

3. A. S. Go et al., "AHA Statistical Update: Heart Disease and Stroke Statistics—2013 Update," *Circulation* 127 (2013): e6–e245.

4. R. C. Colley et al., "Physical Activity of Canadian Adults: Accelerometer Results from the 2007 to 2009 Canadian Health Measures Survey," *Health Reports* 22, no. 1 (March 2011).

5. K. Langlois and D. Garriguet, "Sugar consuption among Canadians of all ages," *Health Reports* 22, no. 3 (September 2011): 23–7.

6. World Health Organization, "Global and Regional Food Consumption Patterns and Trends," www.who.int/nutrition/topics/3_foodconsumption/en/.

7. Centers for Disease Control and Prevention, "Vital Signs: Avoidable Deaths from Heart Disease, Stroke, and Hypertensive Disease United States, 2001–2010," *Morbidity and Mortality Weekly Report* 62, no. 35 (September 6, 2013): 721-7.

8. L. E. Samuels et al., "Coronary Artery Disease in Identical Twins," *Annals of Thoracic Surgery* 68, no. 2 (August 1999): 594–600.

9. A. Evans et al., "The Genetics of Coronary Heart Disease: The Contribution of Twin Studies," *Twin Research* 6, no. 5 (October 2003): 432–41.

10. D. Ornish et al., "Intensive Lifestyle Changes for Reversal of Coronary Heart Disease," *Journal of the American Medical Association* 280, no. 23 (December 16, 1998): 2001–7.

11. Ibid.

12. L. L. Schierbeck et al., "Effect of Hormone Replacement Therapy on Cardiovascular Events in Recently Postmenopausal Women: Randomized Trial," *BMJ* 345 (October 2012): e6409.

13. I. Benakanakere et al., "Synthetic Progestins Differentially Promote or Prevent 7,12-Dimethylbenz(a)anthracene-Induced Mammary Tumors in Sprague-Dawley Rats," *Cancer Prevention Research* 3, no. 9 (September 10, 2010): 1157.

14. M. B. Azad et al., "Gut Microbiota of Healthy Canadian Infants: Profiles by Mode of Delivery and Infant Diet at 4 Months," *Canadian Medical Association Journal* 185 (March 19, 2013): 373–4.

15. R. McCraty, "The Energetic Heart: Bioelectrical Communication Within and Between People," *Clinical Applications of Bioelectromagnetic Medicine* (New York: Markov, 2004), 541–62.

16. M. Franco et al., "Population-wide Weight Loss and Regain in Relation to Diabetes Burden and Cardiovascular Mortality in Cuba 1980–2010: Repeated Cross Sectional Surveys and Ecological Comparison of Secular Trends," *BMJ* 346 (April 9, 2013): f1515.

17. National Center for Health Statistics, "Health, United States, 2012" (Hyattsville, MD: National Center for Health Statistics, 2013).

18. Centers for Disease Control and Prevention, "Prevalence of Coronary Heart Disease—United States, 2006–2010," *Morbidity and Mortality Weekly Report* 60, no. 40 (October 14, 2011): 1377–81.

19. H. Zhang et al., "Discontinuation of Statins in Routine Care Settings: A Cohort Study," *Annals of Internal Medicine* 158, no. 7 (April 2, 2013): 526–34.

20. C. R. Mikus et al., "Simvastatin Impairs Exercise Training Adaptations," *Journal of the American College of Cardiology* 62, no. 8 (August 20, 2013): 709–14.

21. A. A. Carter et al., "Risk of Incident Diabetes among Patients Treated with Statins: Population Based Study," *BMJ* 346 (May 23, 2013): f2610.

22. C. R. Dormuth et al., "Use of High Potency Statins and Rates of Admission for Acute Kidney Injury: Multicenter, Retrospective Observational Analysis of Administrative Databases," *BMJ* 346 (March 19, 2013): f880.

23. M. Gulati et al., "Exercise Capacity and Risk of Death in Women," *Circulation* 108 (September 13, 2003): 1554–9.

24. Mikus et al., "Simvastatin Impairs Exercise Training Adaptations."

25. O. H. Franco et al., "Primary Prevention of Cardiovascular Disease: Cost-effectiveness Comparison," *International Journal of Technology Assessment in Health Care* 23, no. 1 (January 2007): 71–9.

26. R. Rubinshtein et al., "Assessment of Endothelial Function by Non-invasive Peripheral Arterial Tonometry Predicts Late Cardiovascular Adverse Events," *European Heart Journal* 31, no. 9 (May 2010): 1142–8.

27. T. Ugajin et al., "White-coat Hypertension as a Risk Factor for the Development of Home Hypertension: The Ohasama Study," *Archives of Internal Medicine* 165, no. 13 (July 11, 2005): 1541–6.

28. GE Better Health 2010 Study Fact Sheet: Patient-Doctor Disconnect on Healthy Living Revealed (Fairfield, CT: General Electric, 2010).

29. D. M. Tarn et al., "Physician-Patient Communication about Dietary Supplements," *Patient Education and Counseling* 91, no. 3 (June 2013): 287–94.

30. GE Better Health 2010 Study Fact Sheet.

31. C. B. Esselstyn Jr. et al., "A Strategy to Arrest and Reverse Coronary Artery Disease: A 5-year Longitudinal Study of a Single Physician's Practice," *Journal of Family Practice* 41, no. 6 (December 1995): 560–8.

32. A. Tirosh et al., "Changes in Triglyceride Levels and Risk for Coronary Heart Disease in Young Men," *Annals of Internal Medicine* 147, no. 6 (September 18, 2007): 377–85.

33. K. M. Dickinson et al., "Endothelial Function Is Impaired after a High-salt Meal in Healthy Subjects," *American Journal of Clinical Nutrition* 93, no. 3 (March 2011): 500–5.

34. S. M. Ghosh, "Enhanced Vasodilator Activity of Nitrite in Hypertension: Critical Role for Erythrocytic Xanthine Oxidoreductase and Translational Potential," *Hypertension* 61, no. 5 (May 2013): 1091–1102.

35. K. Rahman and G. M. Lowe, "Garlic and Cardiovascular Disease, a Critical Review," *Journal of Nutrition* 136 (2006): 736–40.

36. H. Vasabthi and R. P. Parameswari, "Indian Spices for a Healthy Heart," *Current Cardiology Reviews* 6, no. 4 (November 2010): 274–9.

37. Ibid.

38. G. A. Burdock and I. G. Carabin, "Safety Assessment of Coriander Essential Oil as a Food Ingredient," *Food and Chemical Toxicology* 47 (2009): 22–34.

39. P. M. Lind et al., "Circulating Levels of Persistent Organic Pollutants (POPs) and Carotid Atherosclerosis in the Elderly," *Environmental Health Perspectives* 120, no. 1 (January 2012): 38–43.

40. J. H. Yang et al., "Associations between Organochlorine Pesticides and Vitamin D Deficiency in the U.S. Population," *PLoS ONE* 7, no. 1: e30093.

41. A. E. Mitchell et al., "Ten-Year Comparison of the Influence of Organic and Conventional Crop Management Practices on the Content of Flavonoids in Tomatoes," *Journal of Food Chemistry* 55, no. 15 (July 2007): 6154–9.

42. J. M. de Koning Gans et al., "Tea and Coffee Consumption and Cardiovascular Morbidity and Mortality," *Arteriosclerosis, Thrombosis, and Vascular Biology* 30, no. 8 (August 2010): 1665–71.

43. A. Beresniak et al., "Relationships between Black Tea Consumption and Key Health Indicators in the World: An Ecological Study," *BMJ Open* 2, no. 6 (November 8, 2012).

44. D. P. DiMeglio and R. D. Mattes, "Liquid Versus Solid Carbohydrate: Effects on Food Intake and Body Weight," *International Journal of Obesity* 24, no. 6 (June 2000): 794–800.

45. D. Mozaffarian et al., "180,00 Deaths Worldwide May Be Associated with Sugar Soft Drinks," American Heart Association Meeting, Abstract #MP22 (March 2013).

46. L. de Koning et al., "Sweetened Beverage Consumption, Incident Coronary Heart Disease, and Biomarkers of Risk in Men," *Circulation* 125, no. 14 (April 10, 2012): 1735–41.

47. T. T. Fung, "Sweetened Beverage Consumption and Risk of Coronary Heart Disease in Women," *American Journal of Clinical Nutrition* 89, no. 4 (April 2009): 1037–42.

48. J. Liu et al., "Association of Coffee Consumption with All-Cause and Cardiovascular Disease Mortality," *Mayo Clinic Proceedings* 88, no. 10 (August 2013): 1066–74.

49. H. C. Hung et al., "Fruit and Vegetable Intake and Risk of Major Chronic Disease," *Journal of the National Cancer Institute* 96, no. 21 (November 3, 2004): 1577–84.

50. A Bellavia et al., "Fruit and Vegetable Consumption and All-Cause Mortality: A Dose-Response Analysis," *American Journal of Clinical Nutrition* 98, no. 2 (August 2013): 454–9.

51. P. Ronksley et al., "Association of Alcohol Consumption with Selected Cardiovascular Disease Outcomes: A Systematic Review and Meta-Analysis," *BMJ* 342 (February 2011): d671.

52. K. L. Stanhope et al., "Consumption of Fructose and High Fructose Corn Syrup Increases Postprandial Triglycerides, LDL-Cholesterol, and Apolipoprotein-B in Young Men and Women," *Journal of Clinical Endocrinology & Metabolism* 96, no. 10 (October 1, 2011): E1596–E1605.

53. W. C. Willett et al., "Intake of Trans Fatty Acids and Risk of Coronary Heart Disease among Women," *Lancet* 341, no. 8845 (March 6, 1993): 581–5.

54. John M. Burns, "13-Week Dietary Subchronic Comparison Study with MON 863 Corn in Rats Preceded by a 1-Week Baseline Food Consumption Determination with PMI Certified Rodent Diet #5002," December 17, 2002, cera-gmc.org/docs/decdocs/05-184-001.pdf.

55. R. A. Vogel et al., "Effect of a Single High-fat Meal on Endothelial Function in Healthy Subjects," *American Journal of Cardiology* 79, no. 3 (February 1, 1997): 350–4.

56. B. Prayson, J.T. McMahon, and R.A. Prayson, "Fast Food Hamburgers: What Are We Really Eating?" *Annals of Diagnostic Pathology* 12 (2008): 406-9.

57. R. deShazo, S. Bigler, and L. Skipworth, "The Autopsy of Chicken Nuggets Reads 'Chicken Little'," *American Journal of Medicine* S0002-9343, no. 13 (September 13, 2013): 00396-3.

58. S. Rohrmann et al., "Meat Consumption and Mortality: Results from the European Prospective Investigation into Cancer and Nutrition," *BMC Medicine* 11, no. 63 (March 7, 2013).

59. Harvard School of Public Health, "Eating Processed Meats, But Not Unprocessed Red Meats, May Raise Risk of Heart Disease and Diabetes," news release, May 17, 2010.

60. D. Feskanich, W. Willett, and G. Colditz, "Calcium, Vitamin D, Milk Consumption, and Hip Fractures: A Prospective Study among Post Menopausal Women," *American Journal of Clinical Nutrition* 77, no. 2 (February 2003): 504–11.

61. L. T. ho-Pham et al., "Veganism, Bone Mineral Density, and Body Composition: A Study of Buddhist Nuns," *Osteoporosis International* 20, no. 12 (December 2009): 2087–93.

62. W. H. W. Tang et al., "Intestinal Microbial Metabolism of Phosphatidylcholine and Cardiovascular Risk," *New England Journal of Medicine* 368, no. 17 (2013): 1575–84.

63. J. David Spence, David J. A. Jenkins, and Jean Davignon, "Egg Yolk Consumption and Carotid Plaque," *Atherosclerosis* 224, no. 2 (August 2012): 469–73.

64. A. Fasano, "Zonulin and Its Regulation of Intestinal Barrier Function: The Biological Door to Inflammation, Autoimmunity, and Cancer," *Physiological Reviews* 91, no. 1 (January 2011): 151-75.

65. M. Leenders et al., "Fruit and Vegetable Consumption and Mortality," *American Journal of Epidemiology* 178, no. 4 (2013): 590–602.

66. J. Uribarri et al., "Advanced Glycation End Products in Foods and a Practical Guide to Their Reduction in the Diet," *Journal of the American Dietetic Association* 110, no. 6 (June 2010): 911–6.

67. L. E. Cahill et al., "Prospective Study of Breakfast Eating and Incident Coronary Heart Disease in a Cohort of Male US Health Professionals," *Circulation* 128, no. 4 (July 2013): 337–43.

68. J. D. LeCheminant et al., "Restricting Night-time Eating Reduces Daily Energy Intake in Healthy Young Men: A Short-term Cross-over Study," *British Journal of Nutrition* available on CJO2013. doi:10.1017/S0007114513001359 (May 23, 2013): 1–6.

69. J. E. Brown et al., "Intermittent Fasting: A Dietary Intervention for Prevention of Diabetes and Cardiovascular Disease?" *British Journal of Diabetes & Vascular Disease* 13, no. 2 (March–April 2013): 68–72.

70. M. Hatori et al., "Time-Restricted Feeding without Reducing Caloric Intake Prevents Metabolic Diseases in Mice Fed a High-Fat Diet," *Cell Metabolism* 15, no. 6 (May 17, 2012): 846–60.

71. E. S. George et al., "Chronic Disease and Sitting Time in Middle-Aged Australian Males: Findings from the 45 and Up Study," *International Journal of Behavioral Nutrition and Physical Activity* 10, no. 20 (February 8, 2013).

72. P. T. Katzmarzyk and I. Lee, "Sedentary Behaviour and Life Expectancy in the USA: A Cause-deleted Life Table Analysis," *BMJ Open* 2, no. 4 (July 9, 2012).

73. C. L. Edwardson et al., "Association of Sedentary Behaviour with Metabolic Syndrome: A Meta-Analysis," *PLOS One* 7, no. 4 (April 13, 2012): e34916.

74. J. L. M. Tse et al., "Bus Driver Well-being Review: 50 Years of Research," *Transportation Research Part F: Traffic Psychology and Behaviour* 9, no. 2 (March 2006): 89–114.

75. H. Naci and J. Ioannidis, "Comparative Effectiveness of Exercise and Drug Interactions on Mortality Outcomes: Metaepidemiological Study," *BMJ* 347 (October 2013): f5577.

76. C. Faselis et. al., "Body Mass Index, Exercise Capacity, and Mortality Risk in Male Veterans with Hypertension," *American Journal of Hypertension* 25, no. 4 (April 2012): 444–50.

77. R. H. Fagard and V. A. Cornelissen, "Effect of Exercise on Blood Pressure Control in Hypertensive Patients," *European Journal of Preventive Cardiology* 14, no. 1 (February 2007): 12–7.

78. R. Cade et al., "Effect of Aerobic Exercise Training on Patients with Systematic Arterial Hypertension," *American Journal of Medicine* 77, no. 5 (November 1984): 785–90.

79. K. T. Borer et al., "Two Bouts of Exercise Before Meals, but Not after Meals, Lower Fasting Blood Glucose," *Medicine and Science in Sports and Exercise* 41, no. 8 (August 2009): 1606–14.

80. L. DiPietro et al., "Three 15-minute Bouts of Moderate Postmeal Walking Significantly Improves 24-h Glycemic Control in Older People at Risk for Impaired Glucose Tolerance," *Diabetes Care* 36, no. 10 (October 2013): 3262-8.

81. W. Swardfager et al., "Exercise Intervention and Inflammatory Markers in Coronary Artery Disease: A Meta-analysis," *American Heart Journal* 163, no. 4 (April 2012): 666–76.

82. C.P. Wen et al., "Minimum Amount of Physical Activity for Reduced Mortality and Extended Life Expectancy: A Prospective Cohort Study," *The Lancet* 378, no. 9798 (October 2011): 1244-53.

83. F. B. Hu et al., "Television Watching and Other Sedentary Behaviors in Relation to Risk of Obesity and Type 2 Diabetes Mellitus in Women," *Journal of the American Medical Association* 289, no. 14 (April 9, 2003): 1785–91.

84. G. J. Egger et al., "Estimating Historical Changes in Physical Activity Levels," *Medical Journal of Australia* 175, nos. 11–12 (December 3–17, 2001): 635–36.

85. L. Lanningham-Foster et al., "Labor Saved, Calories Lost: The Energetic Impact of Domestic Labor-saving Devices," *Obesity Research* 11, no. 10 (October 2003): 1178–81.

86. W. E. Kraus et al., "Inactivity, Exercise, and Visceral Fat. STRRIDE: A Randomized, Controlled Study of Exercise Intensity and Amount," *Journal of Applied Physiology* 99, no. 4 (October 2005): 1613–8.

87. M. Papp et al., "Increased Heart Rate Variability But No Effect on Blood Pressure From 8 Weeks of Hatha Yoga," *BMC Research Notes* 6, no. 59 (2013): 1-9.

88. M. Satyapriya et al., "Effect of Integrated Yoga on Street and Heart Rate Variability in Pregnant Women," *International Journal of Gynecology & Obstetrics* 104, no. 3 (March 2009): 218-22.

89. D. Lakkireddy et al., "Effect of Yoga on Arrhythmia Burden, Anxiety, Depression, and Quality of Life in Paroxysmal Atrial Fibrillation: The YOGA My Heart Study," *Journal of the American College of Cardiology* 61, no. 11 (March 19, 2013): 1177-82.

90. O. Devasena and P. Narhare, "Effect of Yoga on Heart Rate and Blood Pressure and Its Clinical Significance," *International Journal of Biological and Medical Research* 2, no. 3 (2011): 750-3.

91. K. Van Proeyen, "Training in the Fasted State Improves Glucose Tolerance during Fat-rich Diet," *Journal of Physiology* 588 (Pt 21) (November 1, 2010): 4289–4302.

92. I. Tabata, et al., "Effects of Moderate-intensity Endurance and High-intensity Intermittent Training on Anaerobic Capacity and VO2max," *Medicine and Science in Sports and Exercise* 28. no. 10 (October 1996): 1327-30.

93. J. Little, et al., "A Practical Model of Low-volume High-intensity Interval Training Induces Mitochondrial Biogenesis in Human Skeletal Muscle: Potential Mechanisms," *The Journal of Physiology* 588 (Pt 6) (March 15, 2010): 1011-22.

94. J. Levine and J. Miller, "The Energy Expenditure of Using a 'Walk-and-Work' Desk for Office Workers with Obesity," *British Journal of Sports Medicine* 41 (2007): 558-61.

95. M. Wilson, et al., "Diverse Patterns of Myocardial Fibrosis in Lifelong, Veteran Endurance Athletes," *Journal of Applied Physiology* 110, no. 6 (June 2011): 1622-6.

96. T. Stalder et al., "Cortisol in Hair and the Metabolic Syndrome," *Journal of Clinical Endocrinology and Metabolism* 98, no. 6 (June 2013): 2573–80.

97. S. Richardson et al., "Meta-Analysis of Perceived Stress and Its Association with Incident Coronary Heart Disease," *American Journal of Cardiology* 110, no. 12 (December 15, 2012): 1711–6.

98. C. A. Jackson and G. D. Mishra, "Depression and Risk of Stroke in Midaged Women: A Prospective Longitudinal Study," *Stroke* 44, no. 6 (June 2013): 1555–60.

99. E. C. Suarez et al., "Depression Inhibits the Anti-inflammatory Effects of Leisure Time Physical Activity and Light to Moderate Alcohol Consumption," *Brain, Behavior, and Immunity* 32 (August 2013): 144–52.

100. L. L. Watkins et al., "Association of Anxiety and Depression with All-Cause Mortality in Individuals with Coronary Heart Disease," *Journal of the American Heart Association* 19, no. 2 (March 2013): e00068.

101. M. Miller et al., "Impact of Cinematic Viewing on Endothelial Function," *Heart* 92 (2006): 261–2.

102. A. B. Bhavanani et al., "Immediate Effect of Sukha Pranayama on Cardiovascular Variables in Patients of Hypertension," *International Journal of Yoga Therapy* 21, no. 1 (September 2011): 73–6.

103. V. Malhotra et al., "Pranayama and Heart," *National Journal of Basic Medical Sciences* 1, no. 1 (July–September 2010): 11–4.

104. A. M. Dabhade et al., "Effect of Pranayama (Breathing Exercise) on Arrhythmias in the Human Heart," *Explore* 8, no. 1 (January–February 2012): 12-5.

105. G. Affleck, "Construing Benefits from Adversity: Adaptational Significance and Dispositional Underpinnings," *Journal of Personality* 64, no. 4 (December 1996): 899-922.

106. R. A. Emmons and M. E. McCullough, "Counting Blessings versus Burdens: An Experimental Investigation of Gratitude and Subjective Well-being in Daily Life," *Journal of Personality and Social Psychology* 84, no. 2 (February 2003): 377-89.

107. R. H. Schneider et al., "Stress Reduction in the Secondary Prevention of Cardiovascular Disease: Randomized, Controlled Trial of Transcendental Meditation and Health Education in Blacks," *Circulation: Cardiovascular Quality and Outcomes* 5, no. 6 (November 2012): 750-8.

108. B. E. Kok et al., "How Positive Emotions Build Physical Health: Perceived Positive Social Connections Account for the Upward Spiral Between Positive Emotions and Vagal Tone," *Psychological Science* 24, no. 7 (July 1, 2013): 1123-32.

109. L. Supaat et al., "Effects of Swedish Massage Therapy on Blood Pressure, Heart Rate, and Inflammatory Markers in Hypertensive Women," *Evidence-Based Complementary and Alternative Medicine* (August 18, 2013): 171852.

110. A. D. Kay et al., "The Effect of Deep-tissue Massage Therapy on Blood Pressure and Heart Rate," *Journal of Alternative and Complementary Medicine* 14, no. 2 (March 2008): 125-28.

111. Friedmann et al., "Animal Companions and One Year Survival of Patients after Discharge from a Coronary Care Unit," *Public Health Reports* 95, no. 4 (July–August 1980): 307-12.

112. J. K. Vombrock and J. M. Grossberg, "Cardiovascular Effects of Human-Pet Interactions," *Journal of Behavioral Medicine* 11, no. 5 (October 1988): 509-17.

113. K. Allen, J. Blascovich, and W. Mendes, "Cardiovascular Reactivity and the Presence of Pets, Friends, and Spouses: The Truth about Cats and Dogs," *Psychosomatic Medicine* 65, no. 5 (September/October 2002): 727-39.

114. S. Hall et al., "Sexual Activity, Erectile Dysfunction, and Incident Cardiovascular Events," *American Journal of Cardiology* 105, no. 2 (January 2010): 192-5.

115. M. Sands-Lincoln et al., "Sleep Duration and Coronary Heart Disease Among Postmenopausal Women in the Women's Health Initiative," *Journal of Women's Health* 22, no. 6 (June 2013): 477-86.

116. C. S. Hung et al., "Mobile Phone 'Talk-Mode' Signal Delays EEG-Determined Sleep Onset," *Neuroscience Letters* 421, no. 1 (June 21, 2007): 82-6.

117. R. B. Weller et al., "UVA Lowers Blood Pressure and Vasodilates the Systemic Arterial Vasculature by Mobilisation of Cutaneous Nitric Oxide Stores," *Journal of Investigative Dermatology* 133, supplement 1 (May 2013): S209-21.

118. R. S. Sneed and S. Cohen, "A Prospective Study of Volunteerism and Hypertension Risk in Older Adults," *Psychology and Aging* 28, no. 2 (June 2013): 578-86.

119. M. E. Pagano et al., "Alcoholics Anonymous–Related Helping and the Helper Therapy Principle," *Alcoholism Treatment Quarterly* 29, no. 1 (January 1, 2010): 23-34.

120. S. Post, "Altruism, Happiness and Health," *International Journal of Behavioral Medicine* 12, no. 2 (2005): 66-77.

121. A. Grant and J. Dutton, "Beneficiary or Benefactor: Are People More Prosocial When They Reflect on Receiving or Giving?" *Psychological Science* 23, no. 9 (September 1, 2012): 1033-39.

122. J. Yogendra et al., "Beneficial Effects of Yoga Lifestyle on Reversibility of Ischaemic Heart Disease: Caring Heart Project of International Board of Yoga," *Journal of the Association ofPhysicians of India* 52 (April 2004): 283-9.

123. S. Arora and J. Bhattacharjee, "Modulation of Immune Responses in Stress by Yoga," *International Journal of Yoga* 1, no. 2 (July–December 2008): 45-55.

124. S. Sinha et al., "Improvement of Glutathione and Total Antioxidant Status with Yoga," *Journal of Alternative and Complementary Medicine* 13, no. 10 (December 2007): 1085-90.

125. C. Wang et al., "Tai Chi on Psychological Well-Being: Systematic Review and Meta-Analysis," *BMC Complementary and Alternative Medicine* 10, no. 23 (May 21, 2010). doi:10.1186/1472-6882-10-23.

126. J. Holt-Lunstad, T. Smith, and J. B. Layton, "Social Relationships and Mortality Risk: A Meta-Analytic Review," *PLoS Medicine* 7, no. 7 (July 27, 2010): e1000316.

127. M. Miyata et al., "Beneficial Effects of Waon Therapy on Patients with Chronic Heart Failure: Results of a Prospective Multicenter Study," *Journal of Cardiology* 52, no. 2 (October 2008): 79-85.

128. T. Kihara et al., "Waon Therapy Improves the Prognosis of Patients with Chronic Heart Failure," *Journal of Cardiology* 53, no. 2 (2009): 214-8.

129. J. Cheng et al., "Acupuncture Therapy for Angina Pectoris: A Systematic Review," *Journal of Traditional Chinese Medicine* 34, no. 4 (December 2012): 494-501.

130. J. Oschman, "Can Electrons Act as Antioxidants? A Review and Commentary," *Journal of Alternative and Complementary Medicine* 13, no. 9 (2007): 955-67.

131. G. Chevalier et al., "Earthing: Health Implications of Reconnecting the Human Body to the Earth's Surface Electrons," *Journal of Environmental and Public Health* (January 2012): epub 291541.

132. G. Chevalier et al., "Earthing (Grounding) the Human Body Reduces Blood Viscosity—a Major Factor in Cardiovascular Disease," *Journal of Alternative and Complementary Medicine* 19, no. 2 (February 2013): 102-10.

133. E. V. Bräuner et al., "Indoor Particles Affect Vascular Function in the Aged: An Air Filtration–based Intervention Study," *American Journal of Respiratory and Critical Care Medicine* 177, no. 4 (February 15, 2008): 419-25.

134. D. Q. Rich et al., "Association Between Changes in Air Pollution Levels During the Beijing Olympics and Biomarkers of Inflammation and Thrombosis in Healthy Young Adults," *Journal of the American Medical Association* 307, no. 19 (May 16, 2012): 2068-78.

135. S. D. Adar, "Fine Particulate Air Pollution and the Progression of Carotid Intima-Medial Thickness: A Prospective Cohort Study from the Multi-Ethnic Study of Atherosclerosis and Air Pollution," *PLoS Medicine* 10, no. 4 (2013): e1001430.

136. Presented at the EuroPRevent 2013 conference: "Long-term Exposure to Fine Particles of Traffic Pollution Associated with Increased Risk of Heart Disease: Results from Large Cohort Study Presented at EuroPRevent 2013," European Society of Cardiology, April 18, 2013.

137. M. Sørensen et al., "Road Traffic Noise and Incident Myocardial Infarction: A Prospective Cohort Study," *PLoS One* 7, no. 6 (2012): e39283.

138. U.S. Department of Health and Human Services "The Health Consequences of Involuntary Exposure to Tobacco Smoke: A Report of the Surgeon General" (U.S. Department of Health and Human Services, Centers for Disease Control and Prevention, Coordinating Center for Health Promotion, National Center for Chronic Disease Prevention and Health Promotion, Office on Smoking and Health, 2006).

139. I. Al-Saleh et al., "Phthalates Residues in Plastic Bottled Waters," *Journal of Toxicological Sciences* 36, no. 4 (August 2011): 469–78.

140. J. L. Carwile et al., "Canned Soup Consumption and Urinary Bisphenol A: A Randomized Crossover Trial," *Journal of the American Medical Association* 306, no. 20 (November 23–30, 2011): 2218–20.

141. P. M. Lind and L. Lind, "Circulating Levels of Bisphenol A and Phthalates Are Related to Carotid Atherosclerosis in the Elderly," *Atherosclerosis* 218, no. 1 (September 2011): 207–13.

142. Al-Saleh et al., "Phthalates Residues in Plastic Bottled Waters."

143. Lind and Lind, "Circulating Levels of Bisphenol A and Phthalates."

144. D. Melzer et al., "Urinary Bisphenol A Concentration and Risk of Future Coronary Artery Disease in Apparently Healthy Men and Women," *Circulation* 125, no. 12 (March 27, 2012): 1482–90.

145. D. Melzer et al., "Association of Urinary Bisphenol A Concentration with Heart Disease: Evidence from NHANES 2003/06," *PLoS One* 5, no. 1 (January 13, 2010): e8673.

146. "Lipstick and Lead: Questions and Answers," U. S. Food and Drug Administration, page last updated June 5, 2013.

147. "Teen Girls' Body Burden of Hormone-Altering Cosmetics Chemicals," Environmental Working Group, September 24, 2008.

148. G. Sarwar et al., "Indoor Fine Particles: The Role of Terpene Emissions from Consumer Products," *Journal of the Air & Waste Management Association* 54, no. 3 (March 2004): 367–77.

149. M. A. Parker et al., "Effect of Cell Phone Exposure on Physiologic and Hemotoligic Parameters of Male Medical Students of Bijapur (Karnataka) with Reference to Serum Lipid Profile," *Journal of Basic and Clinical Physiology and Pharmacology* 21, no. 2 (2010): 201–10.

150. B. Saini, "Effect of Mobile Phone and BTS Radiation on Heart Rate Variability," *International Journal of Research in Engineering and Technology* 2, no. 4 (April 2013): 662–6.

151. A. Alhusseiny, M. Al-Nimer, and A. Majeed, "Electromagnetic Energy Radiated from Mobile Phone Alters Electrocardiographic Records of Patients with Ischemic Heart Disease," *Annals of Medical and Health Sciences Research* 2, no. 2 (July, 2012): 146–51.

152. H. Bauchner, P. B. Fontanarosa, and R. Golub, "Evaluation of the Trial to Assess Chelation Therapy (TACT)," *Journal of the American Medical Association* 309, no. 12 (March, 2013): 1291–2.

153. D. R. Davis et al., "Changes in USDA Food Composition Data for 43 Garden Crops, 1950 to 1999," *Journal of the American College of Nutrition* 23, no. 6 (December 2004): 669–82.

154. "Product Review: Protein Powders and Drinks Review," last modified June 21, 2013, accessed November 11, 2013, www.consumerlab.com/reviews/ Protein_Powders_Shakes_Drinks_Sports_%20Meal_Diet/NutritionDrinks/.

155. "Product Review: Green Tea Supplements, Drinks, and Brewable Teas Review," updated September 27, 2013, accessed November 11, 2013, www. consumerlab.com/reviews/Green_Tea_Review_Supplements_and_Bottled/ Green_Tea.

156. "Product Review: CoQ10 and Ubiquinol Supplement Review," last modified June 13, 2013, accessed November 11, 2013, www.consumerlab.com/reviews/ CoQ10-Ubiquinol-Supplements-Review/CoQ10.

157. "Product Review: Vitamin D Supplements Review," last modified October 4, 2013, accessed November 11, 2013, www.consumerlab.com/reviews/ vitamin_D_supplements_review/Vitamin_D.

158. G.A. Lamas, et al., "Effect of Disodium EDTA Chelation Regimen on Cardiovascular Outcomes in Patients with Previous Myocardial Infarction: The TACT Randomized Trial." *Journal of the American Medical Association* 27, no. 309 (March 27, 2013): 1241-50.

159. K. E. Kelley et al., "Identification of Phthalates in Medications and Dietary Supplement Formulations in the United States and Canada," *Environmental Health Perspectives* 120, no. 3 (March 2012): 379–84.

160. U. Alehagen et al., "Cardiovascular Mortality and N-terminal-oriBNP Reduced Combined Selenium and Coenzyme Q10 Supplementation: A 5-year Prospective Randomized Double-Blind Placebo-Controlled Trial among Elderly Swedish Citizens," *International Journal of Cardiology* 167, no. 5 (September 2013): 1860–6.

161. P. Brøndum-Jacobsen et al., "25-Hydroxyvitamin D Levels and Risk of Ischemic Heart Disease, Myocardial Infarction, and Early Death: Population-Based Study and Meta-Analyses of 18 and 17 Studies," *Arteriosclerosis, Thrombosis, and Vascular Biology* 32, no. 11 (November 2012): 2794–2802.

162. V.K. Santhanakrishnan et al., "A Causal Association between Vitamin D Status and Blood Pressure: A Mendelian Randomization Study in up to 150,846 Individuals," European Society of Human Genetics conference, Abstract #C18.2 (June 2013).

163. W. H. Tang et al., "Intestinal Microbial Metabolism of Phosphatidylcholine and Cardiovascular Risk," *New England Journal of Medicine* 368, no. 17 (April 25, 2013): 1575-84.

164. M. L. Jones et al., "Cholesterol Lowering and Inhibition of Sterol Absorption by *Lactobacillus reuteri* NCIMB 30242: A Randomized Controlled Trial," *European Journal of Clinical Nutrition* 66, no. 11 (November 2012): 1234–41.

Index

A

ACE inhibitors, 39–40
acid reflux medications, 249
A1C tests, 21, 65
acupuncture, 214–215
adenosine triphosphate (ATP), 256
adrenal gland, 26
advanced glycation end products (AGEs),
 20–21, 93, 113, 114, 136–137
Affleck, Glen, 192
air fresheners, 220, 223
air pollution
 indoor, 219–224
 outdoor, 224–226
alcohol, 98
alpha-lipoic acid, 263
Amen, Daniel, 210
anger, 195–197
angina pectoris, 56, 214
angioplasty, 40–42
animal products. *See* meat
antibacterial soap, 236
antibiotics, 108, 111–113, 260
anxiety, 183
apple pie spice, 88
apples, 89
arteries, 16–17, 49
artificial sweeteners, 94, 101
arugula, 85
ashwagandha, 264
asparagus, 96
aspartame, 101
aspirin therapy, 260–261
atrial fibrillation, 168, 177

B

beef production, 108. *See also* meat
beets, 87, 96
bell peppers, 96
belly fat, 153
berberine, 264
beta blockers, 38–39
beverages, 90–95
Bigler, Steven, 109
Bittman, Mark, 115

blenders and juicers, 128–129, 138–139,
 142–143
blood clotting, 153
blood pressure. *See* high blood pressure
blood sugar
 AGE link, 20–21
 exercise effects on, 152
 fasting blood test, 65
 nutrition effects on, 83, 91, 93
 statin drugs effects on, 36
blood tests, 21, 62–67
blood thinners, 43
blood vessels, 16–22, 84
body weight, 152
bok choy, 96
bone health, 114
BPA, 103, 131, 228–231, 232
breakfast, 144–145, 146
breathing techniques, 185–191, 209–210
Broken Heart Syndrome, 180
bypass surgery, 45–48

C

calcium scoring, 57–58
caloric intake, 8–9
cardiac rehabilitation programs, 76–77
carotenoids, 96
carotid intimal medial thickness (CIMT),
 59–60
carrots, 96
carvedilol, 39
casserole dishes, 143
catechins, 90
celery, 87
cell phones, 238–240
chelation therapy, 243
chicken, 114
chips, 104–105
cholesterol
 advanced blood test, 63
 exercise effects on, 152
 as heart disease factor, 14
 medications for, 34–38, 249
 nutrition effects on, 20, 91, 93, 102, 103
 probiotic effects on, 259

external counter pulsation (ECP), 44
eyes, burning, 223

F

fake food, 108–109
Falk, Ehrling, 49
Fasano, Alessio, 119
fast food
    avoiding, 110–111
    harmful effects of, 105–110
fasting, 144–146
fat (dietary), 83, 101, 107–108
Fat, Sick and Nearly Dead (Cross), 128, 138
fatigue, 55–56
ferritin, 66
fish, 116, 117–118
fitness. *See* exercise
flavonoids, 90, 98
food additives, 101–104
food allergies and intolerances, 118–120
food labels, 100–101, 131
food preparation strategies
    cooking, 105, 134, 136–137, 142–144
    kitchen clean sweep, 126–127
    once-a-week prep, 99, 105
    planning ahead, 135
    prescription summary, 268–269
    shopping, 130–131
Forks Over Knives, 86
formaldehyde, 236
Framingham Study, 7
Friedman, Erika, 197
Friedman, Meyer, 181, 217
fruit, fruit juice, 94, 140–141. *See also*
    plant foods

G

garlic, 88, 96
genetically modified organisms (GMOs),
    103–104, 131
genetics, 12–15, 22–25
GGT (blood test), 66
Gibala, Martin, 174
ginger, 88
GI system, 82. *See also* gut bacteria
glycation, 20–21
gratitude, 191–193
greens, 84–87, 98–99
green tea, 41, 90, 264
grocery shopping, 130–131
grounding (Earthing), 202, 215–217

group support, 210–212
Gruentzig, Andreas, 40–41
gut bacteria, 28–29, 82, 259–260
gym memberships, 171–172

H

Hartzler, Geoffrey, 42
HDL cholesterol, 17, 19. *See also*
    cholesterol
health care providers
    communication with, 72–75
    finding, 71–72
    relationship with, 69–71, 74, 76–77
Health Diagnostic Laboratory Inc. (HDL
    Labs), 67
Health Professionals Follow-Up Study, 96
heart attack, 14, 49
heart disease. *See also* screening tools
    contributing factors, 14
    patient statistics, 7–8
    prevalence, 4–5
    prevention, 9–11
    risk factors, 7, 83
    screening for, 6–7
    symptoms, 55–56
heart failure, defined, 14
HeartMath software, 210
heart rate, 185
heart rate variability (HRV), 167–168,
    206, 239
herbal remedies, 201–202
herbs and spices, 87–89, 113, 140
HgbA1C, 21, 65
high blood pressure
    acupuncture for, 214–215
    breathing techniques for, 185–191, 209
    exercise effects on, 151–152, 168–169
    as heart disease factor, 14
    massage effects on, 197
    medications for, 38–40
    nutrition for, 84–87, 96–97
    sodium effects on, 103
    from stress, 182
    sun effects on, 202
    white coat hypertension, 64
high fructose corn syrup, 101, 102, 131
HIIT (high intensity interval training),
    173–175
Hippocrates, 80
holistic health, 15–16, 31
home furnishings, 220, 223
homocysteine, 63, 96

About the Author

Joel K. Kahn, MD, serves as Clinical Professor of Medicine at the Wayne State University School of Medicine and Director of Cardiac Wellness at Michigan Healthcare Professionals. He also holds teaching positions at Oakland University William Beaumont Medical School (Associate Professor) and the University of South Florida (Lecturer) and has lectured at major medical conferences around the nation.

A summa cum laude graduate of the University of Michigan School of Medicine, Dr. Kahn completed a residency in Internal Medicine in Ann Arbor, receiving both the clinical and research excellence awards. His cardiology fellowship was completed at University of Texas Southwestern Medical Center in Dallas and Interventional Cardiology training was at Saint Luke's Mid America Heart Institute in Kansas City under the leadership of Drs. Geoffrey Hartzler and Barry Rutherford.

A founding member of the International Society of Integrative, Metabolic and Functional Cardiovascular Medicine, Dr. Kahn is the first physician in Michigan to be certified by the Society of Heart Attack Prevention and Eradication and the first in the world to be certified in metabolic cardiology by the University of South Florida and the American Academy of Anti-Aging Medicine. He has written more than 150 medical articles, book chapters, and monographs and has served on several editorial boards of medical journals.

Dr. Kahn has been selected for Top Doc awards for many years. He serves on an advisory wellness board for the Daniel Plan at Saddleback Church and has served as chairman of his local American Heart Association and March of Dimes. He also writes the "Holistic Heart Doc" column for *Reader's Digest* magazine. He enjoys music of all kinds, yoga, kayaking, paddleboarding, and playing with his rescue dogs Jake and Eva. Married with three children, Dr. Kahn has been practicing cardiology in the Detroit area for more than 20 years.

Reader's digest

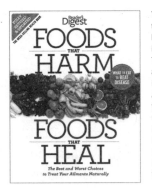
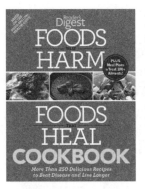
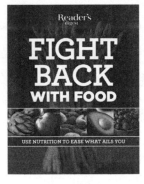
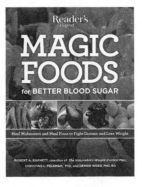